PRAISE FOR *THE HOLISTIC DENTAL MATRIX*

"As an author of seven books on wellness and an alternative eye doctor, I have seen many cases where serious eye pathology is related to a dental issue. Dr. Nick Meyer's book The Holistic Dental Matrix *is the book I have been looking forward to. It has valuable information on the importance of dental health and the link to dental health to our general well-being and health. This book will be a valuable addition to my library and I will recommend it to all of my patients!"*

-Edward Kondrot, MD, MD(H), CCH, DHT
Past President, Arizona Homeopathic and Integrative Medical Association

"Dr. Nicholas Meyer is truly one of the most enlightened Holistic Dentists in the USA and we are fortunate that he has shared his story and insights in this very easy to read book that he has artfully written. I feel fortunate practicing in a community where Dr. Meyer lives so that I can refer my patients to him. I'm doubly glad that he's written this book that my patients can read so they can see why I'm sending them for the referral. Dr. Meyer has done a great service in explaining a subject in very readable fashion that needed explaining in a way that patients can appreciate and easily understand."

-Dr. Bruce H Shelton, MD, MD(H), DiHOM FBIH
Homeopathic Family Physician
Past President, AZ Homeopathic and Integrative Medical Association

"Thank you for all the time and effort you expended to help so many in so many ways. You've earned stars in heaven. You are great!"

-Doris Rapp, MD, MD(H)
Practitioner, Researcher, Author

"Every now and then someone comes along who proves they are ahead of their time. Dr. Meyer's brilliant and timely work in The Holistic Dental Matrix *shows this to be true with a well thought out and structured approach to bringing the mouth and the body together. Dr. Meyer's* The Holistic Dental Matrix *is long overdue and is an excellent guide to understanding a facet of dentistry many dentists are ill-informed and/or misinformed on, and which too many have prematurely and unnecessarily and unfortunately dismissed as irrelevant."*

-Lee Ostler, DDS
Past President, American Academy for Oral Systemic Health (AAOSH)

"Dr. Nicholas Meyer provides a layman's guide to non-invasive dental approaches that can help people regain control of their health. Using non-technical language, he helps the reader learn the underlying causes of their ill health and how this relates to their dental problems. Dr. Meyer also describes dental products and resources that can promote good health. This book is a must read for those who wish to empower themselves to greater wellness."

-Todd Rowe, MD, MD(H), CCH, DHt
Founder, American Medical College of Homeopathy

"Dr. Meyer shows the rare ability to see things from many perspectives. He has been practicing for years but hasn't stopped learning, thinking and incorporating new ideas into his daily professional life. He has singlehandedly expanded our understanding of cavitations and MARCoNS. I look forward to working with him to bring the MARCoNS/NICO data to publication soon."

-Ritchie Shoemaker, MD
Researcher & Author

"The Holistic Dental Matrix *is the 21st Century informational guide to oral health. Renowned dentist, Dr. Nicholas Meyer, makes holistic dentistry simple to understand and follow. Dr. Meyer follows the lead of Dr. Hal Huggins and documents the mounting evidence against toxins like mercury and fluoride. He offers practical solutions on holistic treatments and therapies. I loved this book and will recommend it to all of my patients."*

-Jack Wolfson, MD
The Paleo Cardiologist

"The Holistic Dental Matrix *is an excellent resource for dental patients seeking to educate themselves about one of the most important yet commonly neglected parts of the body, impacting overall health and well-being. Too often, subtle dental or head and neck problems are neglected due to lacking awareness that Dr. Meyer's book,* The Holistic Dental Matrix, *provides. For this reason, Dr. Meyer should be congratulated for doing a great job helping to save lives and spare people's needless expense, distress and disease."*

-Leonard G. Horowitz, DMD, MA, MPH, DNM, DMM (hon.)
Editor-in-chief, *Medical Veritas*

"We are all indebted to Dr. Nick Meyer for his efforts in producing this critical, detailed book on dentistry, The Holistic Dental Matrix. *I know from my 58 years of medical practice that every health challenge will be easier to solve if patients have access to the potential life-saving information found in this book and choose to follow the recommendations it makes. Everyone needs a copy of this amazingly comprehensive book in order to better understand the vital contribution a healthy mouth can make to achieving optimal health and longevity."*

-G.F. Gordon MD, DO, MD(H.)

"After reviewing this great book and watching Dr. Meyer in action I can vouch for the veracity of the information that Dr. Meyer presents here in The Holistic Dental Matrix. *His diagnostic acumen and surgical skills are a great combination that gives tremendous credibility to this book."*

-Nishant Chauhan, DMD, MPH, MBA
Dental Anesthesiologist

"This very readable, truly enjoyable and immensely significant endeavor on behalf of the health of the dental patient is cogently written. In my opinion every dentist should definitely keep this book on the bookshelf alongside The Web that has No Weaver: Understanding Traditional Chinese Medicine (TCM) *by T.J. Kaptchuk, OMD."*

-Dr. Norman Thomas, DDS, BDS (Hons) PhD
Chancellor, International College of Craniomandibular Orthopedics (ICCMO)

"Dr. Nick Meyer has written an important document that will advance the health of all of humanity. Written for the layman so that they understand the historical forces that molded the practice of dentistry in the United States, Dr. Meyer traces his own evolution through the biologic and holistic mine field. Because he persevered and dedicated his practice to this very subject, and more importantly, learned to apply that knowledge to treat heretofore 'untreatable' cases, Dr. Meyer has given millions hope for healthy longevity. I highly recommend this book to all dentists and all other health practitioners who are looking to widen their scope of practice to include enhanced patient care."

-Dr. Bill Williams, DMD
Solstice Dental Advisors

"Your book is brilliant, Nick—it is well written and clear."

-Martha Grout, MD, MD(H) President,
Arizona Homeopathic and Integrative Medical Association

"Dr. Meyer has done a wonderful presentation in this new book. The importance of dental health is generally overlooked by physicians who fail to recognize the distal ramifications of irritations and infections in the jaw and teeth. Of drastic influence are the mercury amalgams which must be removed in all cases of chronic disorders. I recommend all health enthusiasts to read this book; it will no doubt leave a lasting impression."

-Prof. [Dr. of Med.] Charles McWilliams
Grand Master - Sacred Medical Order • Church of Hope

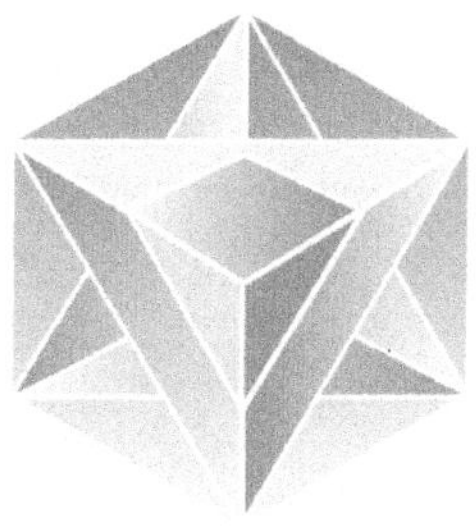

What Is This Symbol?

The Merkaba (or Merkabah) is a tool and technique that facilitates humans to reach their full potential in any and all areas of their life. The most important thing about the Merkaba is the connection to one unified universal mind called the omnipresence (God) and the awareness that we are creators of our own world and can create anything. (Courtesy of Jean Sheehan & Millennium Education)

The Merkaba is my favorite ancient symbol and resonated with me to be present within this book. I can see how the structural integration can take place through these interconnected planes and points. The points being the outward signs that are made manifest of the internal conditions within our body.

THE HOLISTIC DENTAL MATRIX

How Your Teeth Can Control Your Health & Well-being

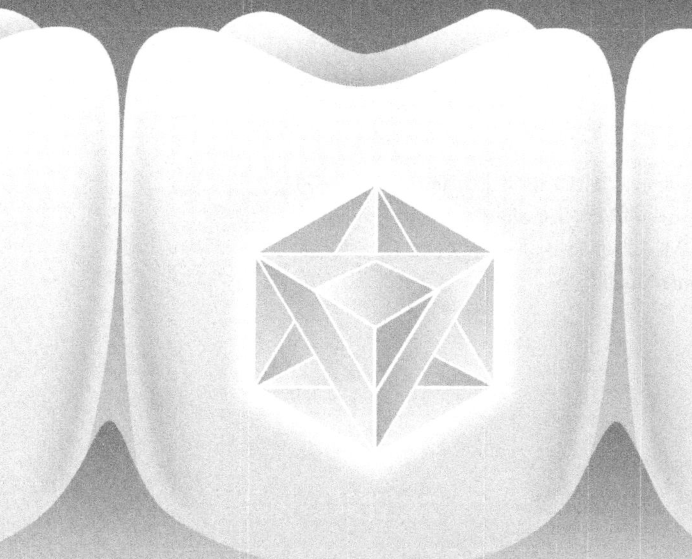

Nicholas J. Meyer, DDS, DNM

Foreword by Burton Goldberg

Printed in the United States of America

First Printing, 2016

ISBN: 978-1-546-56041-8

Millennium Management
5705 N. Scottsdale Rd, Bldg D Suite #110
Scottsdale, AZ 85250

The Holistic Dental Matrix™
Multi-Dimensional Dental Paradigm™

www.DrNicholasMeyer.com

Cover art, design of Matrix Charts, and book layout by Tom Ardans and Don Schreer of Schreer Design Inc, with the 'Merkabah' icon provided by James Levin, MD, and his wife Natalie.

DEDICATION

To my wife Nancy, my greatest inspiration.
For without her
This would not have been given life
And my children and grandchildren – my cheerleaders

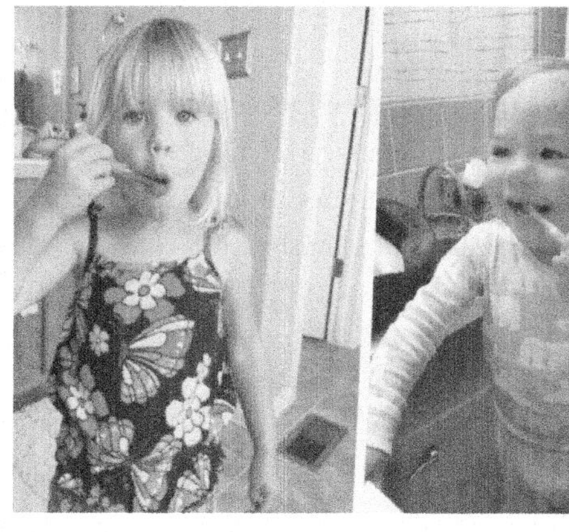

ACKNOWLEDGEMENTS

This endeavor has touched many lives on its way to creation. I am especially thankful for the help that I have received from Susan Wright, writer and editor, who helped me stay focused on the writing and completion and who gave form to the words on paper; Dr. James Levin, whose editorial eye and guidance helped forge a crisp and sharp document; my lay reviewers, Donna Willis, Vic Gonda and Marissa Russo; and my professional reviewers, who helped me see how truly important this book is to the world.

INVITATION

Please opt-in on our website: www.DrNicholasMeyer.com and like our Facebook page to join our community. The website contains additional important information and opportunities to learn more across a wide and diverse field of interest in holistic dentistry. Individual chapters are also available for purchase on the website: www.DrNicholasMeyer.com.

DISCLAIMER

This book is for educational purposes only. It is written for members and prospective members of The Millennium Management, an ecclesiastical private expressive association, by its director, Nicholas J Meyer, a pastoral health practitioner and counselor. Under this appointment, Dr. Meyer is an ordained minister and chaplain who ministers to the sick and suffering under international law and under Arizona statute Sec. 32-3271.(3)

Any similarities to real individuals are purely coincidental. The privacy of those whose stories are told is held a sacred trust. Their stories are all on file and in my possession.

LEGAL NOTICE

The information in this book is not intended to diagnose nor treat any disease or condition that you or a loved one may be suffering. It is not a sub statute for examination, diagnosis and medical/dental care provided by a licensed and qualified health care professional. Do not attempt to treat yourself, your child or anyone else without proper medical/dental supervision. This book is written under the authority of God as my maker and not under the color of law as held by any governmental agency. I am ordained minister of the Sacred Medical Order of the Church of Hope.

I stand on the grounds of the organic Constitution of these United States. I claim my rights to Freedom of Religion (1st Amendment); Freedom of Speech (9th Amendment) as well as the ability to express my views in public.

DISCLAIMER OF LIABILITY

The materials in the book are provided to you "as is" without warranty of any kind, either expressed or implied, including, but not limited to the implied warranties or merchantability, fitness for a particular purpose, or non-infringement.

In no event shall Nicholas Meyer, his staff, heirs, assigns, the Sacred Medical Order of the Church of Hope, or Millennium Dental Associates or its associates or employees be liable for any damages or incidental damages or damages for loss of profits, revenue, use, or data, whether brought in contract or tort arising out of or connected with this book or the use, reliance upon, or performance of any material contained in or accessed from this book or our website.

Your reading of this book implies that you agree to the release of liability noted above.

The physicians and or physician dentists at Millennium Landmark, a Private Expressive Association, treat members with whatever they consider to be the most effective agent or modality even if it is not standard-of-care medicine/dentistry. This includes traditional medical/dental concepts, Tennant Biomodulator, chiropractic acupuncture concepts, herbal medicine, essential oils, homeopathics, hyperbaric, nutrition, frequencies, infrared sauna, ozone, etc.

There is adequate case law within our land that clearly sets forth the principles so stated herein. Civil courts have no power or jurisdiction to determine the regularity or validity of the judgment of a church tribunal expelling a member from further communion and fellowship in the church. Membership in a church creates a different relationship from that which exists in other voluntary societies formed for business, social, literacy or charitable purposes.

In writing this book, I am not writing as a D.D.S. I am writing as a licensed pastoral health practitioner and counselor and under Arizona statute section 32-3271 and under my 1st and 9th Amendment rights of the United States Constitution.

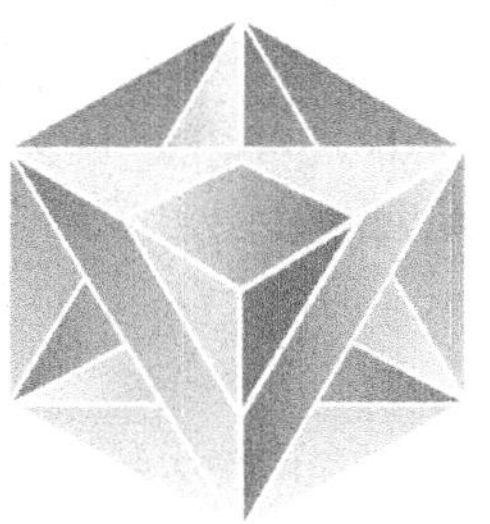

HUMPTY DUMPTY AND HOLISTIC MEDICINE

By Dr. Nicholas J. Meyer

Humpty Dumpty sat on a wall
Humpty Dumpty had a great fall
All the kings' horses and all the kings' men
Couldn't put Humpty together again

But a few old Druids thought, "Hey, why not?"
So gathered up Humpty they did on the spot
Off to the depths of the realm they did go
With herbs and spices and energies aglow

They figured out how Humpty's do heal
And soon they found the real deal
The eggshell hard cover had cracked all about
But transmutation they said with a shout

So energy lights and scalar waves
Aimed ever so carefully at the major craze
Blended the cracks back into a whole
Humpty came back to life, from death he was stole

They got good ole Humpty back up on that wall
And all the kings' horses and all the kings' men
Carted off those wise Druids who knew how to mend
And burned all their books so their story would end

The tale continues on into this age
Modern day Druids you'd say are a sage
With potions and gizmos at their disposal
Good folk all around praise their Godly proposals

The story's the same, yes even today
The king's still in power and Humpty must pay
Some books have been found, the Druids had hid
That mend all the people that give them their bid

When a Druid steps out of the king's finely drawn lines
The king he doth strike hard, their hands do they bind
With sanctions and fines these Druids are saddled
Unable to heal when oh so embattled.

Under cover of darkness they must ply their trade
'Cause the kings of today, say they must forbade
These brilliant new Druids still find a way
Their talents and knowledge are here to stay

Humpty Dumpty and Holistic Medicine

TABLE OF CONTENTS

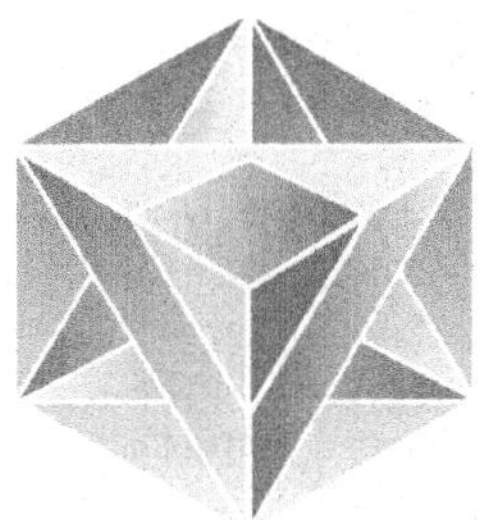

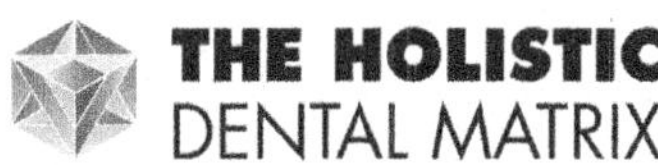

Look up your symptoms in the left column, then find the appropriate chapters to read.

▼ If your symptom is... go to Chapter ►	Mercury Amalgam	Fluoride & Other	TMD	Airway	Periodontal	Cavitations & Bone Disease	Root Canal	Missing & Malposed Teeth	Dental Materials (no Hg)	Lyme	Mold Toxicity CIRS
	2	3	4	4	6	5	5	4	6	4,6	6
Adrenal Disease									•		
Brain									•		
Fog	•										
Stroke				•				•			
Cognitive impairment	•	•		•				•	•	•	•
Trouble concentrating				•							•
Dementia				•							
Memory problems				•							•
Cells											
Mitochondrial dysfunction	•	•		•		•	•		•		
Ear Problems & Postural Imbalances											
Hissing, buzzing, ringing or roaring sounds (tinnitus)	•		•					•			
Diminished hearing (subjective hearing loss)	•		•					•			
Ear pain without infection (otalgia)			•					•			
Clogged, stuffy, itchy ears, feeling of fullness			•					•			
Balance problems (vertigo or disequilibrium)	•		•					•			•
Emotional & Behavioral									•		
Irritability, anxiety, nervousness, difficulty breathing	•	•		•				•	•		
Restlessness	•			•				•			
Exaggerated response to stimulation	•										
Emotional instability	•			•				•			
Loss of self confidence	•							•			
Shyness or timidity	•							•			
Lethargy/drowsiness	•			•							
Insomnia	•			•							
Despondency	•										
Depression & anxiety				•							
Slower reaction times				•							

Look up your symptoms in the left column, then find the appropriate chapters to read.

▼ If your symptom is... go to Chapter ►	Mercury Amalgam 2	Fluoride & Other 3	TMD 4	Airway 4	Periodontal 6	Cavitations & Bone Disease 5	Root Canal 5	Missing & Malposed Teeth 4	Dental Materials (no Hg) 6	Lyme 4,6	Mold Toxicity CIRS 6
Emotional & Behavioral (cont.)											
Confusion											•
Disorientation											•
Decreased learning of new knowledge											•
Word recollection issues											•
Mood swings											•
Eye Pain & Orbital Problems											
Pain, above, below, behind			•					•			
Bloodshot eyes (hyperemia)			•					•	•		•
Bulging appearance (exophtalmia)			•					•			
Pressure behind the eyes (retro-orbital pain)			•					•			
Light sensitivity (photophobia)			•					•			•
Watering of the eyes (lacrimation)		•	•					•			•
Drooping of the eye lid (ptosis)			•					•			
Visual impairment	•										
Glaucoma	•										
Restricted, dim vision	•										
Blurred vision											•
Disorders				•							
GI-gastrointestinal									•		
Food sensitivity, especially milk & eggs	•										
Abdominal cramps	•	•									•
Colitis, Crohn's Disease, IBS	•			•							
Diverticulitis	•										
Diarrhea											•
Chronic diarrhea/constipation	•	•									
Dysbiosis	•										
Therapy resistant parasites	•										
Colon cancer	•										
GERD			•	•				•			
Nausea		•									
Loss of appetite		•									

THE HOLISTIC DENTAL MATRIX

Look up your symptoms in the left column, then find the appropriate chapters to read.

▼ If your symptom is... go to Chapter ►	Mercury Amalgam	Fluoride & Other	TMD	Airway	Periodontal	Cavitations & Bone Disease	Root Canal	Missing & Malposed Teeth	Dental Materials (no Hg)	Lyme	Mold Toxicity CIRS
	2	3	4	4	6	5	5	4	6	4,6	6
Head Pain, Headache Problems, Facial Pain											•
Forehead (frontal)	•		•	•				•	•	•	
Temple (temporal)	•		•	•				•	•	•	
"Migraine" type headache	•		•	•				•	•	•	
"Cluster" headache	•		•	•		•		•	•	•	
Under eyes (maxillary sinus headache)			•	•		•		•	•	•	•
Posterior back of head (occipital headache)			•	•				•	•	•	
Hair +/or scalp painful to touch (parietal headache)			•	•				•	•	•	
Trigeminal Neuralgia						•	•				
Heart									•		
Rhythm, abnormal/tachycardia	•			•		•			•		
Atrial fibrillation				•							
EKG, Altered	•			•		•					
Triglycerides, elevated unexplained	•			•							
Cholesterol, elevated unexplained	•			•							
Blood pressure, abnormal	•			•		•					
Cardiomyopathy	•			•							
Coronary heart disease	•			•		•		•			
Mitral valve prolapse	•										
Jaw And Jaw Joint (TMD) Problems											
Clicking, popping jaw points			•	•				•			
Grating sounds (crepitus)			•	•				•			
Jaw lacking, open or closed			•	•				•		•	
Pain in cheek muscles			•	•				•		•	
Uncontrollable tongue, or jaw movement			•	•				•		•	
Kidney											
Chronic kidney disease									•		
Nephritic syndrome	•										
Receiving dialysis	•										
Kidney infection	•										
Cancer					•						

THE HOLISTIC DENTAL MATRIX

Look up your symptoms in the left column, then find the appropriate chapters to read.

▼ If your symptom is... go to Chapter ►	Mercury Amalgam 2	Fluoride & Other 3	TMD 4	Airway 4	Periodontal 6	Cavitations & Bone Disease 5	Root Canal 5	Missing & Malposed Teeth 4	Dental Materials (no Hg) 6	Lyme 4,6	Mold Toxicity CIRS 6
Mouth, Face, Cheek, & Chin Problems			•	•							
Discomfort			•	•				•			
Limited opening (Hypomobility)			•	•				•			
Inability to open smoothly or evenly			•	•				•			
Jaw deviates to one side when opening			•	•				•			
Inability to "find bite"			•	•				•			
Tissue pigmentation, amalgam tattoo	•								•		
Leukoplakia	•										
Stomatitis	•								•		
Ulceration of gums, palate, tongue	•	•							•		
Burning sensation with tingling of lips, face	•								•		
Herpes Simplex I		•				•					
Neck & Shoulder Problems											
Lack of mobility-reduced range of movement		•	•	•				•		•	
Stiffness		•	•	•				•		•	
Neck pain (cervicalgia)			•	•				•		•	
Tired, sore neck muscles			•	•				•		•	
Shoulder aches			•	•				•		•	
Back pain, upper and lower			•	•				•		•	
Arm & finger tingling, numbness +/or pain	•		•	•				•		•	•
Teeth & Gum Problems											
Clenching, grinding at night or day (Bruxism)	•		•		•			•			
Looseness +/or soreness of back teeth			•		•			•			
Tooth pain (toothache)			•		•			•			
Alveolar bone loss	•		•		•			•			
Salivation, excessive	•										
Foul breath	•				•						
Metallic taste	•										•
Bleeding gums	•				•						
Osteoporosis					•						
Discolorations	•	•		•							

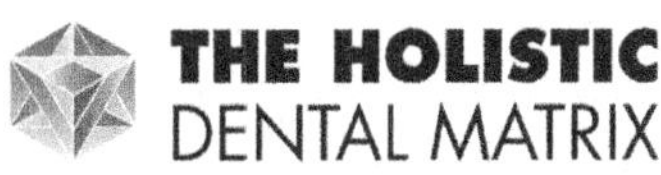

Look up your symptoms in the left column, then find the appropriate chapters to read.

▼ If your symptom is... go to Chapter ►	Mercury Amalgam	Fluoride & Other	TMD	Airway	Periodontal	Cavitations & Bone Disease	Root Canal	Missing & Malposed Teeth	Dental Materials (no Hg)	Lyme	Mold Toxicity CIRS
	2	3	4	4	6	5	5	4	6	4,6	6
Nervous System									•		
Depression, mental	•							•		•	
Depression, manic	•									•	
Numbness & tingling, feet, fingers, toes, lips	•									•	
Muscle weakness progressing to paralysis	•										
Ataxia	•										
Trembling of hands, feet, lips, eyelids, tongue	•	•						•			•
Lack of coordination	•							•			
Myoneural transmission failure, resembling	•										
Myasthenia Gravis	•										
Unexplained sensory symptoms, pain	•					•					
Unexplained numbness or burning sensations	•										
Unusual excitement (ADD/ADHD)		•		•							
Cognitive dysfunction				•						•	•
Panic attacks				•						•	
Memory problem				•						•	•
Systemic Effects									•		
Anemia, unexplained	•										
Fatigue, general	•			•		•				•	•
Loss of appetite w/ or w/o weight loss	•	•									
Loss of weight	•	•									
Hypoglycemia	•										
Allergies	•										
Dermatitis, severe	•	•									
Dermatitis mild-moderate											•
Cold, clammy skin, esp. hands & feet	•										
Multiple chemical sensitivity	•					•				•	
Pre-term low birth weight babies					•						
Pain & achy bones		•									•
Faintness		•									
Metabolic syndrome				•	•	•	•				

THE HOLISTIC DENTAL MATRIX

Look up your symptoms in the left column, then find the appropriate chapters to read.

▼ If your symptom is... go to Chapter ►	Mercury Amalgam	Fluoride & Other	TMD	Airway	Periodontal	Cavitations & Bone Disease	Root Canal	Missing & Malposed Teeth	Dental Materials (no Hg)	Lyme	Mold Toxicity CIRS
	2	3	4	4	6	5	5	4	6	4,6	6
Systemic Effects (cont)											
Insulin resistance (Diabetes)				•	•						
Morning stiffness											•
Obesity				•							
Impotence				•							
Fibromyalgia				•							
Throat Problems											
Swallowing difficulties (dysphagia)			•					•			
Tightness of throat			•					•			
Sore throat without infection (coryza)			•					•			
Voice fluctuations			•					•			
Laryngitis			•					•			
Frequent coughing or constant clearing of THROAT			•					•			
Feeling of foreign object in throat			•					•			
Tongue pain (glossalgia)			•					•			
Salivation (intense)		•	•					•			
Pain in the hard palate, posterior aspect			•					•			
Thyroid									•		
Disturbance	•	•									
Subnormal body temperature	•	•									
Social/lifestyle Intrusions											
Daytime sleepiness				•							
Medication & surgical complications increase				•							
Automobile crashes				•							
Workplace performance impairment				•							
Strained relationships	•		•	•		•	•	•		•	•

FOREWORD

By Burton Goldberg,
The Voice of Alternative Medicine

I first met Dr. Meyer years ago when I ran a cancer clinic in Arizona. I will never forget a case of a prostate cancer that we discerned through electro-dermal screening, a method of determining which pathogen, toxin, parasite, virus, or bacteria is causing a patient's health problems. The patient suffered from excruciating pain in the area of his prostate. Dr. Meyer determined that a tooth that sat on the same meridian as the prostate was causing the pain. The minute Dr. Meyer extracted the tooth the man's pain disappeared.

In America, medical doctors are taught to specialize. Consequently, the various fields of medicine are fragmented and separate from each other. Conventional doctors do not treat the human body as if it functions as a whole. In reality, the human body is intricately connected. There is no better example of this point than the way in which your teeth can control your health and well-being. Most people, including most dentists, are unaware of the connection between the health of their teeth and the health of their bodies. That is why I am thrilled that Dr. Meyer has written *The Holistic Dental Matrix.* It is a book that will revolutionize the way people think about dentistry. It will help you understand how biologic dentistry not only improves the health of the mouth, but also is able to eliminate some of the worst diseases of our time.

The old song that the knee bone is connected to the thigh bone is very true. Every organ of your body is connected by the meridian system and the nervous system. In fact, in Germany dentists are required to be medical doctors—that illustrates the importance of this concept. I learned in Germany that 95 percent of women with breast cancer have a dental involvement. 95 percent! Heart problems, stroke, cancer—all organ malfunctions can be connected to the teeth. Quite often people will have organs removed when they should really have removed the tooth affecting that particular organ.

As Dr. Meyer points out in this book, an acquaintance of mine named Don Margolis, the founder and chairman of the Repair Stem Cell Institute, is another example of how biological dentistry can resolve health problems that at first glance seem unrelated to oral health. Don didn't have cancer, but he was losing a lot of weight, so I sent him to a holistic physician who recommended that Don see a biological dentist. Don ignored that advice and continued to grow worse. He was eating 1,500 calories a day, but was still losing about 2 pounds a week. Three different conventional doctors tried to treat the problem, but the weight loss continued. Don started at 176 pounds and his weight dropped to 123 pounds. Finally, Don decided to listen to the holistic physician's advice. He had the proper dental work done by a biological dentist and he started gaining weight. Today, he's back to a normal weight.

Not only are conventional dentists ignorant that every tooth in the mouth is connected to every system in the body—they're also ignorant of the damage caused by mercury fillings. They're still using mercury fillings to this day. The mercury fillings arrive at the dentists' offices in a container labeled "biohazard." Dentists are not allowed to put the mercury in the sewer system, yet they're putting it in your mouth. Something is radically wrong with that.

When you read Dr. Meyer's book, you will be astounded at the important role that the oral cavity plays in overall health. He is a wealth of information on this topic, sharing his clinical experience in biological dentistry. This book includes a convenient chart that shows exactly which teeth are connected to specific health problems. Not only should every patient read this book—every dentist should also read it since it will change the way they view their profession and allow them to help their patients in a more profound way than they ever have before.

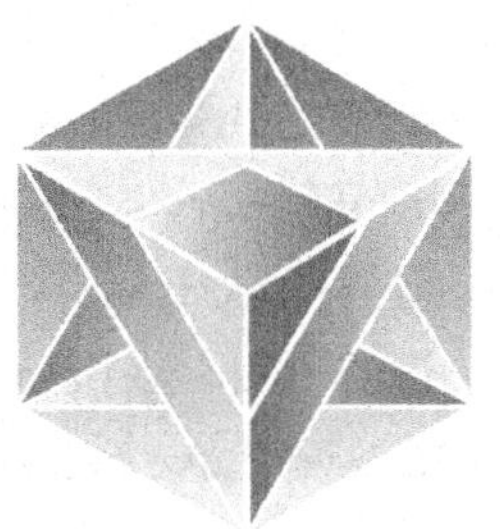

CHAPTER 1

INTRODUCTION, MY STORY

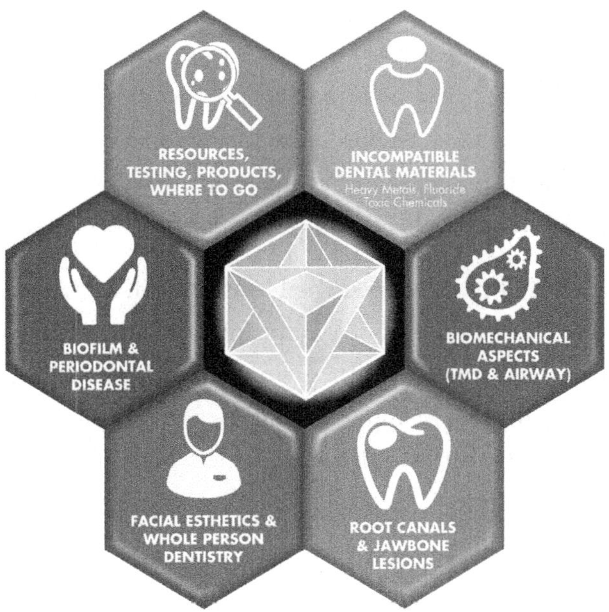

Welcome to the Holistic Dental Matrix™. It's a concept, a way of thinking about your health that you may never have considered before. This model has been developed over my 37+ years of practice.

My early years of practice were pretty much the same as everyone else's. Dentistry was for me a very black and white discipline with few shades of grey. As my world view expanded, and this certainly included dentistry, I've learned that I can't just treat the symptoms of one's dental issues; I have to follow the symptoms in order to find the real problem. Every part of our body works together, and the various aspects of our health can't be isolated.

So when there's a breakdown in one part of your body, it affects your other systems, tissues and organs. This means that your dental issues don't just have an effect on your teeth and mouth; they can also cause health problems all over your body. My appreciation for this developed over many decades.

That's why I've developed the Holistic Dental Matrix, to help you find your way. This book is meant to be used as a guidepost or a handbook to good health, giving you information on holistic dentistry that you can apply to your own life. I want to help you make sense of your symptoms and their possible dental causes and relationships.

The Holistic Dental Matrix is a concept and format for thinking about symptoms, diseases, and health challenges that can be caused, furthered or treated by dental conditions or treatments by a dentist. I created the chart of the Holistic Dental Matrix to assist you in your journey. Find your symptoms on the chart and then see which chapters of the book correspond to you so that you can consult them in order to shed the light of awareness and understanding on the potential causes of your health challenges.

In short, the matrix will help you to take better control of your health care.

For example, say you have a chronic daily headache. With the Holistic Dental Matrix chart, you look under the Health Issue column to find your symptom, then track sideways to find the column with a chapter number in it. That will show you what kind of condition you may have and the corresponding chapter where I discuss the condition and possible solution(s).

Headaches could be caused by a bite imbalance, so you would go to Chapter 4 – TMD and Airway Disorders: I Haven't Got Time for the Pain to find out more about how your misaligned teeth could be causing your chronic headaches. You can also find out how this condition can be treated in a holistic way.

Another example is if you have low energy and brain fog. This could be an indication of incompatible dental materials, so to find out more you go to Chapter 2 – Heavy Metal… And Not the Rock Band Kind! There you find out about materials that can have a detrimental effect on your health. You'll also see in the Holistic Dental Matrix that low energy and brain fog could be an indicator of bone disease, so you can also consult Chapter 5 – Root Canals & Jaw Bone Lesions: Hidden Causes of Disease. There you will discover how disease in your jaw bone can cause adverse reactions throughout your body.

I suggest you start your exploration of this book by looking at the Holistic Dental Matrix in the front of this book or in the Index at the back of this book. To get the most benefit from the matrix, take a moment to step back and visualize your body. Look inside yourself and visualize swirling around within you are the symptoms and conditions that affect your life. Close your eyes, take a breath, and now consider what you are seeing is simply an orchestra of many moving parts and those parts together make up your body. You are the conductor leading the orchestra. You are the one who can notice that something is off.

You can scan the whole to pinpoint the aberration, just like the conductor of an orchestra can hear if the one of the violinists is off.

Using the Holistic Dental Matrix is just like that. You are the conductor, and it's up to you to constantly scan your body. When you feel something is not right, look to the Holistic Dental Matrix. Find the sign or symptom that you're experiencing and proceed to that chapter to see what might be going on with your body. The purpose is to guide you into thinking of a different, bigger picture.

In this book, I will also provide resources for good dental health, and share how to find a holistic dentist who can impact your entire body with their dental treatment, not just your dental symptoms. There's also a chapter on healthy eating because what you eat has a big impact on your dental health. Furthermore, your mouth is the beginning of your digestive process.

I've come to believe that the practice of traditional dentistry doesn't often look far enough beyond the immediate concern to see how your problems are affecting your body as a whole. I support treatments that take into account your entire body, and are as non-invasive and beneficial as possible. I also know that the materials we put into our bodies can have a toxic effect on us, so I suggest products that will benefit your body rather than harm you.

I've seen the advantage that you can get from holistic dentistry after a long career of ongoing study and direct patient care. This book is my attempt to share that knowledge with you, so you can reclaim your life and health.

My Introduction to Holistic Dentistry & Medicine

I began my dental career in 1979, after graduating from Loyola University School of Dentistry in Chicago, Illinois. Dental school was rigorous, yet even while I was training in traditional dentistry, I was interested in looking at new ways of doing things. In my senior year, I was able to participate in a clinical research project on a novel delivery system, the use of sustained time release antibiotics to treat periodontal disease. The findings were published in the *Illinois Dental Journal.*[1] I've always had a drive to share what I've learned, so based on this research, I returned to my undergraduate university, Lewis University in Illinois, to give a lecture on oral microbiology to the microbiology class.

During my senior year, I also entered the Block Drug company essay contest and I won 1st Place with my paper titled

"Dental Students' Role in Community Affairs." Subsequently I then entered this project with the American Association of Public Health Dentistry, and I captured 3rd place in the national competition. The topic, of being involved in community affairs, is an important one to me, and I've been active in community service for much of my life. This includes organizations from the Boy Scouts to the Rotary Club, as well as through speaking to students about dental health and providing free dental screenings for adults and children. It's important to give back because I believe we are all interconnected through our community, in much the same way the systems within our body are interconnected.

That's one reason why I put private practice on hold after I graduated, and I entered the correctional system as a practicing dentist at a maximum security prison in Illinois. It was an eye-opening world for me as I had to walk through half a dozen iron gates to get into my dental office. But it turns out that my two years working in prisons in Dwight and Pontiac, Illinois, provided me with a wealth of human life stories from both inside and outside the walls of the prison.

For a young dental professional, the prisons provided a rich environment in which to stretch my wings and begin my work. The diverse set of residents (prisoners) came with a plethora of dental issues, and I was often the first dentist they had ever seen. I listened to their stories and quickly realized that their dental issues had as much to do with their lives as with their teeth. Based on my work with the prisoners, I returned to Loyola University and gave a presentation on working as a dentist in a correctional facility to encourage other dentists in training to take advantage of the same opportunity that I'd had.

After working in the prisons, I spent almost two years in private practice in Chicago. My practice consisted of the basic procedures characteristic of dentistry: cleaning, fillings, extractions and false teeth. It was pretty standard fare. But even as a young professional, I knew there was more to dentistry because of the wide range of issues that I had encountered in the prison system.

My introduction into the world of holistic dentistry came when I entered private practice in the little farming town of Neoga, Illinois in 1983. The Neoga practice that I purchased provided orthodontia, so I pushed myself to learn as much as I could because I was keenly interested in the area of TMD (temporomandibular joint disturbances) and orthodontia. In fact, I took the last one of the first series of orthodontia courses the weekend prior to my wedding to my wife Nancy—as of the writing of this book, we've just celebrated 33 years of marriage, and I am still taking courses!

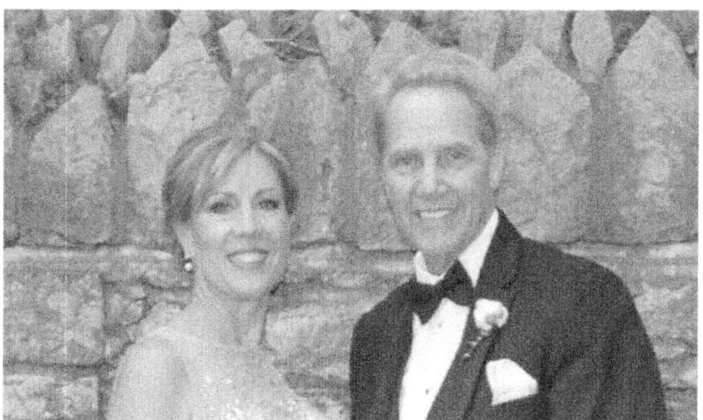

My wife Nancy and me in a recent photo

So, here's the story of how I got involved in holistic dentistry. An employee in my Neoga practice was the first turning point that sent me down the path to becoming a holistic dentist. She unfortunately developed Multiple Sclerosis (MS). At the time I didn't know anything about it other than the name, but she became so sick that she had to leave my practice. A few months later, she came back with a request that I remove her mercury fillings, under a rubber dam, in a particular sequence, and replace them with a certain gold alloy composition determined by some method that was unknown to me.

She brought in a thick sheave of papers from a holistic physician practicing in Las Vegas that discussed why these things would be beneficial. These papers described a whole different way of not only looking at teeth, but also thinking about teeth as a bellwether of your body. Included was a chart that depicted certain relationships of each tooth to other body organs. *WOW*, I thought. *This is really interesting.* It was called a Meridian Chart and planted a seed that grew into a plant that still grows strong in me today. This Meridian Chart, I found out later, connected teeth (which are considered organs in the German biological medicine model) to the internal organs of our body, emotions, skeletal system and more through meridians, which are a set of pathways in the body along which vital energy flows. Keep in mind this was prior to much being known or heard of about acupuncture and the meridians associated with it.

I didn't understand it but I complied with the wishes of my former employee. The doctor whose papers she brought to me haunted me for many years as I referred back to them. They were evidence that there was another way of looking at dentistry, a way that considered how your teeth related to the other areas of your body. It lit a spark inside of me that has burned and consumed my whole life.

You can see an interactive version of the Meridian Chart that shows the relationship of each tooth to your organs at the end of Chapter 1 or use the QR code below.

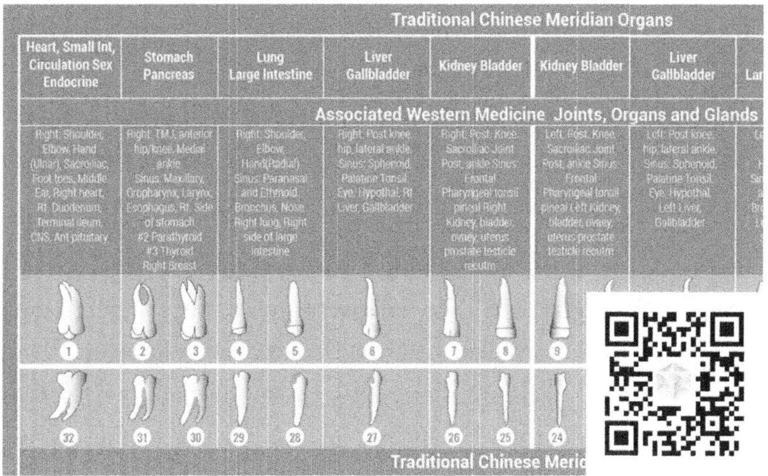

Meridian chart showing the relationship of each tooth to your organs, adaptation by Drs. Louisa Williams and Dietrich Klinghardt. An interactive chart is available on my website: follow QR code.

This experience with my former employee also turned me away from the use of mercury fillings. A seminar leader from Phoenix,

Arizona said at one of the many meetings I attended around that time that maybe mercury fillings weren't such a good idea, and he explained how toxic mercury is to our bodies. That fertilized the seed that was planted by my former employee to shun mercury and learn the best techniques in removing old mercury fillings.

My second turning point came from an unlikely place—a postcard came in the mail from a dental manufacturing company, Myotronics, regarding a training course in orthodontics using a TENS unit to treat temporomandibular disorders (TMD) which are problems often caused by a bad bite. This course promised to give me the missing piece to TMD by showing how important it was to also treat the muscles of your face, jaw and neck. Myotronics recommended that the muscle treatment for TMD is a transcutaneous electric nerve stimulator or TENS unit. Little did I know at the time that this course would be the first step of immersing myself in this discipline for a lifetime to come.

The doors to higher learning had been opened and I eagerly stepped through. I was a relatively new practitioner, being challenged by notions that were so different to everything that I had just learned at Loyola. Yet these early encounters with what I now call holistic dentistry set the stage for my practice in ministering to those in need who have chronic pain disorders of various types.

By 1988, my family had grown to include two beautiful daughters and we moved to Phoenix, AZ. I wanted to have a larger practice area in a more sunny location. It was shortly after our move that I was able to witness and experience holistic medical treatment first-hand on a member of my family.

It started when my little girl, who was then four years old, developed a horrific rash on her body. The doctors were stumped by what was causing it. We applied every preparation we could find, hoping it would stop the itch. Well, that was just wishful thinking. God had another plan for us.

Fortunately I had just joined a Rotary club and one of the speakers was Dr. Konrad Kail, a Naturopathic Physician. I took my daughter to see him, and he used a device called a Computron to analyze her system. He diagnosed an allergy to chlorine. These were mostly new concepts and ideas to me. A Computron is a "bio-energetic" device that picks up alterations in the energy pattern of the body. Interestingly enough, about 4 months prior I had been introduced to this technology at a TMD course I attended.

You see, we had just moved into a condominium in Phoenix and our unit was the closest to the Jacuzzi spa. For two little girls coming out of the frigid plains of Illinois, they thought they had died and gone to heaven. They played for hours in that little spa. We didn't think anything of it. But within a couple of months of regular exposure, the bumps erupted and they were painful and itchy.

Dr. Kail put my daughter on a high strength Vitamin C liquid. This almost immediately stopped the reactivity and itching. Once that was controlled, he "desensitized" her using the Computron device and what is called "Natural Allergy Elimination Technique." Then he created a "remedy." *What the heck is a remedy?* I thought. It turned out it was a little glass vial that she wore in her sock for about an hour, and she was also instructed to stay away from the offending spa for 25 hours. By golly, this did the trick. The allergy never came back.

This experience proved to me that traditional medicine has its limits, and that it helps to look beyond the expected to find a cure. My second experience with holistic medicine was even more serious. A couple of years later, my wife was stricken with shingles. I had only heard of this in school and had not ever actually seen it. Well, I got to see it *big* time. It affected Nancy's mid-face region and included her eye in its advancing path. Nothing we did could stop it.

Then a girl friend of hers offered to take her to a doctor, but she had to be sworn to secrecy. Nancy couldn't tell anyone what she was going to see or experience. It sounded scary, but we were desperate so she went to see the doctor. She came home with a little bottle of drops that looked like water. This was her "remedy." She was to take it religiously for the next couple of days and then get rechecked by her doctor. Fortunately, the virus was stopped in its tracks by this treatment. If it hadn't worked, she would have lost her right eye within a few days.

The clincher of the trifecta however was another life altering event. My youngest daughter once again proved to be a powerful teacher. All was well for a few years until, like a lightning bolt, my baby turned from a lively little girl of about 13 into the living dead. She complained of fatigue much more than sports and school should warrant. Then the crash! She began sleeping 20-22 hours a day. *What in the world!?* we wondered. At first we thought it was a weird passing bug but as the days wore on and on, there was no improvement.

Back to Dr. Kail we went. He used his little box (EAV) device once again and then he rendered his analysis. He found the signature of Epstein Barr virus and Cytomegalovirus—the hall mark signals of Chronic Fatigue Syndrome. The treatment now was different than before. Immediately we began infusions of IV Vitamin C (IV-C). The first day showed no overt response, but then there was movement. We had another IV-C and much greater improvement. We had planned a holiday to see friends in Mexico and there was no way she could go as she was. But I realized that my friend could help once we were in Mexico. So off we went, my little girl in tow, down but not out. While there, we had two additional rounds of IV-C in our room, thanks to my friend. That did it. She was back. My little girl came rebounded with all of her youthful exuberance. We had won this battle.

This was my baptism by fire, and these experiences had a profound effect on me as a medical practitioner. I've seen holistic medicine help the people I love.

I've also had experiences with my own body that have shown me how interconnected our systems are, and how the health of one part of my body impacts on the health of other parts of myself. I've especially seen it during times of psycho-emotional stress. For example, during the various moves that I have made, my back has gone out. At first I thought it was simply a biomechanical reaction, and that I was doing too much physical labor. But despite being very careful, it happened again and again.

The straw that broke the camel's back was when I bent over to throw a little scrap of paper into the trash bin beneath the sink in our home. I fell to the floor and didn't stand up straight for two days. Acupuncture came to my rescue.

That got my attention! I knew that this incident had to be more than a biomechanical occurrence happening within my body. So I set out on a journey to explore my inner self and find out who I really am and what I am about. I realized that I am the product of my childhood, growing up the oldest of seven children in a large Catholic family from Chicago. In order to survive the chaos of my highly energetic family, I withdrew like a turtle into a shell.

To unlock the old chains, my inner work has spanned years and has yielded an inner peace that is magical. In hindsight, the experiences that I went through were preparing me for what I do today when I care for the sick.

You can go to www.DrNicholasMeyer.com to see my video of how holistic dentistry can help with chronic disease. Here's a direct link:

Conclusion

Little was known about holistic practices when I first started my exploration at the beginning of my dental career, but there were many people working within the field and I've been fortunate to benefit from their experiences. Throughout my professional life, I've had an almost insatiable need to learn, integrate and put into practice what I've learned. I came to learn about energy medicine, acupuncture principles, drug therapies, and more. I would go back to my practice armed with new insights and I honed my craft. I never bought into the idea of using drugs as a routine staple for chronic pain management because I was seeing too many cases respond positively without drugs, so I shunned them almost from the start.

My playground may be the mouth and teeth but I can assure you that there is so much more to it. Some of my patients have been kind enough to share their stories of how their dental issues impacted the rest of their health, and they offer encouragement for others who find themselves in need.

My journey has brought me here, so I can share what I have learned with you. I have lectured internationally now for 15 years on the interrelatedness of your dental health and physical health. *The Holistic Dental Matrix* is my attempt to distill into a layman's guide a way to look at your symptoms, and give you hope for a greater level of health and better well-being in your life.

Today at my practice, Millennium Dental Associates, we strive to bring the best and most up to date information in our care of you. To see more on this, go to:

End Note

[1] Meyer, N. "Use of Sustained Time Release Antibiotics in the Treatment of Periodontal Disease." *Illinois Dental Journal* 48.7 (1979).

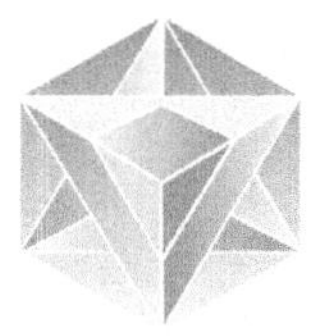

DENTAL ACUPUNCTURE MERIDIAN CHART

By Drs. Louise Williams and Dietrich Klinghardt

RIGHT TEETH UPPER

Traditional Chinese Meridian Organs				
Heart, Small Int, Circulation Sex Endocrine	Stomach Pancreas	Lung Large Intestine	Liver Gallbladder	Kidney Bladder
Associated Western Medicine Joints, Organs and Glands				
Right: Shoulder, Elbow, Hand (Ulnar), Sacroiliac, Foot toes, Middle Ear, Right heart, Rt. Duodenum, Terminal ileum, CNS, Ant pituitary	Right: TMJ, anterior hip/knee, Medial ankle. Sinus: Maxillary, Oropharynx, Larynx, Esophagus, Rt. Side of stomach #2 Parathyroid #3 Thyroid Right Breast	Right: Shoulder, Elbow, Hand(Radial) Sinus: Paranasal and Ethmoid. Bronchus, Nose. Right lung, Right side of large intestine	Right: Post knee, hip, lateral ankle. Sinus: Sphenoid, Palatine Tonsil. Eye. Hypothal, Rt Liver, Gallbladder	Right: Post. Knee. Sacroiliac Joint Post, ankle Sinus: Frontal Pharyngeal tonsil pineal Right Kidney, bladder, ovaey, uterus prostate testicle recutm
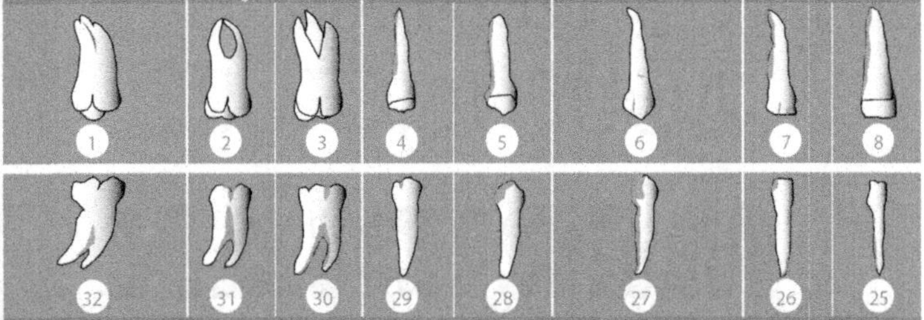 1	2 3	4 5	6	7 8
32	31 30	29 28	27	26 25
Traditional Chinese Meridian Organs				
Heart, Small Int, Circulation Sex Endocrine	Lung Large Intestine	Stomach Pancreas	Liver Gallbladder	Kidney Bladder
Associated Western Medicine Joints, Organs and Glands				
Right: Shoulder, Elbow, Hand (Ulnar), Sacroiliac, Foot toes, Middle Ear, Right heart, Rt. Duodenum, Terminal ileum, CNS,	Right: Shoulder, Elbow, Hand(Radial) Sinus: Paranasal and Ethmoid. Bronchus, Nose. Right lung, Right side of large intestine	Right: TMJ, anterior hip/knee, Medial ankle. Sinus: Maxillary, Oropharynx, Larynx, Esophagus, Rt. Side of stomach #28 Ovaries, Testes, Right Breast	Right: Post knee, hip, lateral ankle. Sinus: Sphenoid, Palatine Tonsil. Eye. ovaries, testes, Rt Liver, Gallbladder	Right: Post. Knee. Sacroiliac Joint Post, ankle Sinus: Frontal Pharyngeal tonsil pineal Right Kidney, bladder, ovaey, uterus prostate testicle recutm

RIGHT TEETH LOWER

LEFT TEETH UPPER

Traditional Chinese Meridian Organs				
Kidney Bladder	Liver Gallbladder	Lung Large Intestine	Stomach Pancreas	Heart, Small Int, Circulation Sex Endocrine
Associated Western Medicine Joints, Organs and Glands				
Left: Post. Knee. Sacroiliac Joint Post, ankle Sinus: Frontal Pharyngeal tonsil pineal Left Kidney, bladder, ovaey, uterus prostate testicle recutm	Left: Post knee, hip, lateral ankle. Sinus: Sphenoid, Palatine Tonsil. Eye. Hypothal, Left Liver, Gallbladder	Left : Shoulder, Elbow, Hand(Radial) Sinus: Paranasal and Ethmoid. Bronchus, Nose. Left lung, Left side of large intestine	Left : TMJ, anterior hip/knee, Medial ankle. Sinus: Maxillary, Oropharynx, Larynx, Esophagus, Left Side of stomach #15 Parathyroid #14 Thyroid Left Breast	Left Shoulder, Elbow, Hand (Ulnar), Sacroiliac, Foot toes, Middle Ear, Left heart, Left Duodenum, Terminal ileum, CNS, Ant pituitary
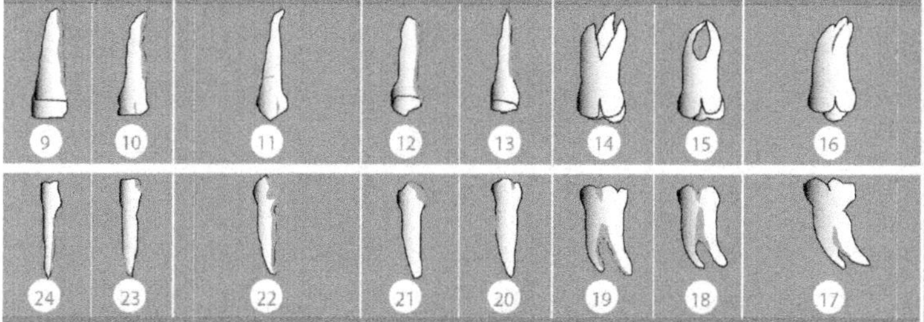 9 10	11	12 13	14 15	16
24 23	22	21 20	19 18	17
Traditional Chinese Meridian Organs				
Kidney Bladder	Liver Gallbladder	Stomach Pancreas	Lung Large Intestine	Heart, Small Int, Circulation Sex Endocrine
Associated Western Medicine Joints, Organs and Glands				
Left: Post. Knee. Sacroiliac Joint Post, ankle Sinus: Frontal Pharyngeal tonsil pineal Left Kidney, bladder, ovaey, uterus prostate testicle recutm	Left: Post knee, hip, lateral ankle. Sinus: Sphenoid, Palatine Tonsil. Eye. ovaries, testes, Left Liver, Gallbladder	Left : TMJ, anterior hip/knee, Medial ankle. Sinus: Maxillary. Oropharynx, Larynx, Esophagus, Left Side of stomach #21 ovaries, testes, Left Breast	Left : Shoulder, Elbow, Hand(Radial) Sinus: Paranasal and Ethmoid. Bronchus, Nose. Left lung, Left side of large intestine	Left Shoulder, Elbow, Hand (Ulnar), Sacroiliac, Foot toes, Middle Ear, Left heart, Left Duodenum, Terminal ileum, CNS, Ant pituitary

LEFT TEETH LOWER

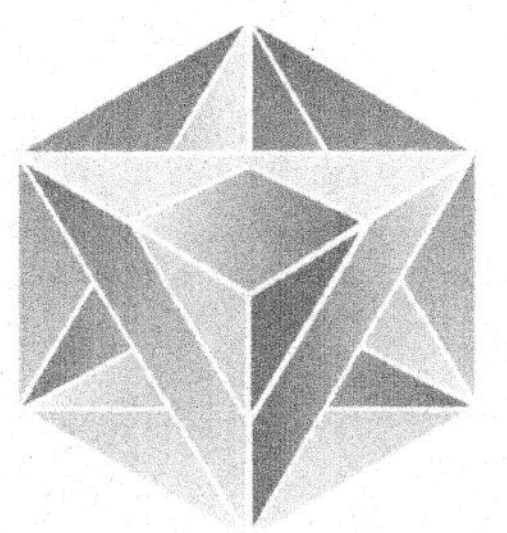

CHAPTER 2

HEAVY METAL... AND NOT THE ROCK BAND KIND!

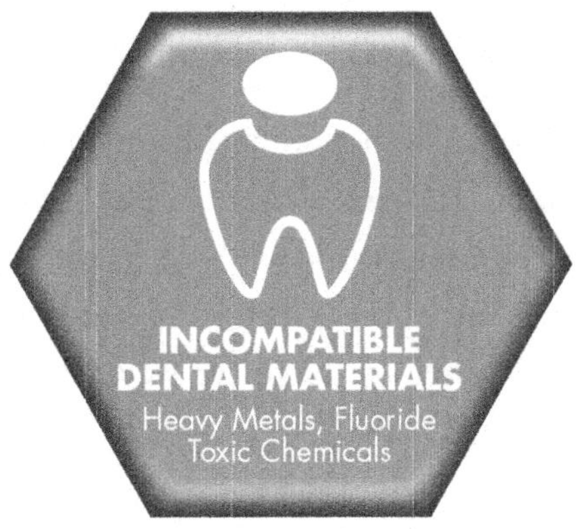

You may not know it, but heavy metals can cause or be related to a large number of symptoms in your body, as outlined in my Holistic Dental Matrix™. What symptoms are you having? It could be emotional or behavioral concerns such as irritability, insomnia or lethargy. Or you might be suffering from physical problems like digestive disease, headache, eye pain or kidney disease. There are also systemic issues like hypoglycemia and faintness, or nervous system disorders such as numbness, tremors or lack of coordination.

All of these things can be caused by common metals used in dentistry. Many heavy metals, such as zinc, copper, chromium, iron and manganese, are essential in tiny amounts. But if these metals accumulate in your body, it can poison you. The most common heavy metals associated with poisoning are lead, mercury, arsenic and cadmium.

We seldom think much about the materials that our dentist uses because we know they've been given the seal of approval by the American Dental Association. So we take it on faith that these things are okay to use in our mouth. And some of them are.

But the dark side is that some dental materials have been found to be unsafe in clinical trials. This is especially true in the context of the toxic world we live in today. Years ago we had less air pollution, food pollution and water pollution, so our bodies weren't as stressed by the toxins we did encounter and the demands of a modern lifestyle.

That's all changed today. We are a race of walking wounded and some of us are just barely treading water to keep from falling into chronic illness. The materials used in your dental work could be adding to your problems… or even causing them!

So what is a metal? By definition a metal is an element that can freely transfer electrons, which means that a current can pass through it. Some metals are better at this than others, but all metals with free electrons can give them up and pass a current. This makes them particularly volatile in how they interact with the tissues in our body. It is this ability that allows the metals to become bio-active or have a greater reactivity in your cells. The metal can actually change how the chemistry of the cell functions. So when there is an alteration of the normal function, it is called a dysfunction.

In this chapter, I'll go over some of the dangers of heavy metals and the most common diseases and symptoms caused by metals like mercury, titanium and nickel. This is an important part of my Multi-Dimensional Dental Paradigm™ that outlines the connection between good health and holistic dentistry.

Mercury Fillings – Is There A Problem? You Decide.

The most common question I hear in my holistic dentistry practice is: "What do I need to know about my silver fillings, and what should I do about them?"

First, you need to know that silver amalgam fillings are about 50 percent mercury. Mercury is a heavy metal that is among the most neurotoxic elements on earth. That means mercury can damage your nervous tissues; not only your brain cells but all of your nervous system which conveys the signals from your brain to the rest of your body.

There is no safe level of mercury for the human body. This means that it is harmful at all doses. One atom of mercury can disable one whole enzyme molecule.

Regarding dentistry, the Environmental Protection Agency (EPA) says that any scraps of filling material have to be treated like a toxic substance, whether the scraps come from creating a new mercury filling or from removing an old filling.[1] It's hard to believe, but according to our government the only safe place to store mercury fillings is in a human being!

ADA's stance

So why are mercury fillings allowed when mercury is known to be toxic?

When the American Dental Association (ADA) was sued years ago over this, they stated they had no duty of care to the public or individuals when it came to amalgam filling material.[2] That's because the ADA is a trade organization that exists solely for the benefit of member dentists. It isn't intended to serve the best interests of the general public.

According to the ADA, mercury amalgam fillings are "manufactured" by the dentist at the time of use and so that makes *the dentist* the responsible party. The ADA does certify that the mercury is mercury and that the alloy powder is what it is said to be. But the mixed product—the "amalgam" that is placed in your tooth, is made by the dentist. The doctor, in their office must mix the certified mercury with the certified alloy powder and that produces the uncertified mercury amalgam filling material. So it's not something that the ADA has to put their seal of approval on. It seems strange that they certify other mixed products used in a dental office, mixed by the dentist at the time of use, but not the mercury amalgam.

And to make matters worse, the ADA Health Foundation owned two patents for amalgam fillings that include mercury

(#4,018,600 & #4,078,921).[3] Is it any wonder the ADA supports the use of mercury amalgam? Also of interest is that the ADA sells the ADA Seal of Acceptance for use on amalgam bottles to cozy relationships with amalgam sellers who "donate" to ADA programs. The ADA also endorses a brand of amalgam separators through its for-profit subsidiary, ADA Business Enterprises.

Today it's estimated, by the insurance industry, that about half of the dentists in the U.S. are no longer using amalgam fillings. The fact that mercury fillings are on the wane is more from natural attrition than any altruistic notions. The newer doctors have a much wider array of restorative (filling) products today than they did generations prior to the 1980s. With so many newer and more cosmetic alternatives, the use of amalgam is just fading away.

That is, unless of course you happen to be locked into an insurance plan that will only pay for mercury amalgam. Also, some low-income state plans will only provide mercury amalgam fillings even though there are other materials that don't contain mercury.

There are political reasons why amalgam is still being used today. FDA hearings and investigations have been held for decades at the demand of consumers, but it wasn't until 2007 when the FDA lost a lawsuit that dental amalgam was finally classified. That's when the FDA declared that mercury amalgam is a Class II substance that is safe for use by everyone.[4]

After filing a number of petitions calling for either a formal ban of amalgam use, or at least placement in FDA's Class III status, the International Academy of Oral Medicine and Toxicology filed a lawsuit in 2014 citing that the FDA has failed to respond within a reasonable time.[5] Placing dental mercury into Class III status would require additional restrictions for vulnerable people, more stringent proof of safety, and an Environmental Impact Statement.

Health Effects

Mercury in your metal fillings is continually being released. It is released at a greater rate and amount when your teeth grind together or against hard substances when you chew, have acidic beverages or food, or have hot food or liquids. That releases mercury vapor which is then inhaled or absorbed right through the tissues of your mouth. The effect can be worse if two mercury fillings are grinding against each other.

For years the dental profession has claimed that the mercury is bound up in the filling and it does not leak out. Perhaps with the science back in the day when amalgam was first used that statement couldn't be challenged because there was no way to refute it. Today however, it has been conclusively shown that mercury does "leak out" from a filling from the moment it is inserted.

One man who has spent decades studying mercury poisoning is Sam Queen, from Colorado Springs, CO. As a health care educator, certified nutrition specialist and investigative medical reporter, Queen has gathered together the signs and symptoms of mercury poisoning. The tabulations he created from his data are incorporated in the body of the Holistic Dental Matrix.[6]

It's an undisputed fact that mercury is a toxin that affects your body—not only your brain and nervous system are impacted, but also your cardiovascular and immune system.

Mercury is stored in fat cells. That may not sound too bad, but did you know the brain is primarily fat? Our brain is only 3 percent of our body by weight, and it uses 25 percent of our body's energy, so it's constantly using a high amount of energy from the rest of our body. Also, all of the nerves of the body are coated in fat for insulation. Owing to the high fat content of the brain and nerves, it's easy to see how our brain can be like a mercury sponge.

When mercury hits your brain, it causes neurons to deteriorate and then short circuit. Neurons are nerve cells that process and transmit information through electrical and chemical signals. The University of Calgary filmed the effects of mercury on neurons, and you can see how a low level of mercury caused the neuron fibers to shrink at an alarming rate.[7]

Our body is remarkable at self-repair, but nothing can stand up to a relentless assault. After a while, your cells can't keep up and fatigue sets in. At some point the structure and function of your body breaks down and then we see what we call a disease. And this isn't just happening in the brain—your organs have nerves as well as your nervous system which links your body together. This shows up in different ways in different people and at varying rates. Hence, this is why there is so much confusion and bafflement for not only the sufferer but also the doctors.

It has been long stated that mercury is locked into the fillings within the teeth and never leaves. However, it was conclusively proven by the University of Calgary's sheep studies that this was not true. A series of these studies were done in 1989 and 1990 when researchers at the University of Calgary Medical School placed radioactive mercury amalgam fillings in sheep's teeth. When the sheep were tested, little mercury was found in their blood and urine, which are the recommended tests for mercury exposure today, while much higher amounts were found in the kidneys.[8] The studies demonstrated the dispersal, distribution and relative amount of the mercury in the subjects' bodies. It also depicted how quickly and thoroughly mercury lodges elsewhere in your body.

The critics of this work made obvious slurs about humans not chewing like sheep—which is true enough. Nonetheless, the real take-home message is that mercury leaves fillings fairly quickly and is carried through your body to target organs that have a lot of fat. Along with your brain, your gut has a lot of fat. Your gut has been called the home to our microbiome or "second brain" which controls your immune system. So it's no wonder that people with mercury exposure are having immune problems as well as tingling and coordination issues.

Metals, like mercury, that are foreign to your body cause what is known as metalloproteins to develop. These are substances that become the targets of the immune system and are in part responsible for the development of autoimmune illness. When the mercury interacts with the normal proteins in your body, your immune system sees these proteins as foreign and tries to remove them. Unfortunately, since the mercury-bound molecule is so similar to the "normal" protein, the normal protein also becomes a target for the immune system.

Mercury Exposure

There are other ways you can ingest mercury, which adds to the toxic levels stored in your body. Mercury can also accumulate in your body from eating tuna, which contains a higher level of mercury than in many other fish. It is also found in higher concentrations in planktonic life forms and water cleaners like shrimp and lobster. When aquatic life forms eat mercury, there's no way for them to "detox" their little body. So the mercury sits there waiting to later be eaten by you.

So how does mercury get in the water? Most of it comes from industrial waste. One of the greatest sources of water contamination is from coal burning and related pollution. When the hundreds of power plants burning coal in China and elsewhere release their toxic clouds into the air, it gets taken up into the atmosphere and then falls out of the sky in rain. There are no national boundaries when it comes to weather. A similar effect takes place with the soil. The rains wash down the particles that are in the atmosphere onto the land where crops are grown. The plants take up the mercury and we then ingest it without even knowing it. Dental office waste has been measured to contribute around 12 percent of the mercury load in industrial waste as measured in studies carried out in San Francisco and Seattle.

If you are old enough, you may recall when Mount St. Helens of Washington State erupted. This eruption spewed millions of tons of debris into the atmosphere for miles around. This debris contained not only the annoying ash that covered everything but also a whole boatload of toxic substances. So it isn't very hard to visualize that the affected zone took on a great dose of both harmful and non-harmful elements. Those who farm the land had no choice but to continue as if nothing had happened.

Beauty products can also contain mercury. It's not allowed for products manufactured here in the U.S., but with the Internet and global travel, people are increasingly getting hold of cosmetics that were manufactured in other countries.

There are also beauty products you put on or near your mouth that contain a variety of metals such as lead, bismuth, titanium oxide (whitening and reflective agent), and cadmium (red) in cosmetics and sunscreens.

TESTIMONY BY E.S.

My medical doctor recommended that I see Dr. Meyer to do the work (mercury amalgam removal) in order to help restore my health. One year later, my allergies have decreased 90 percent. I no longer take allergy medication; also my hair is thick and healthy and finally growing long and my immune system has returned to normal. Thank you Dr. Meyer, for all that you have done for me.

Safe Treatment

The way to stop mercury exposure from your dental amalgam fillings is to have your fillings safely removed. You can replace your old fillings with a variety of substances such as: 98 percent gold alloy, resin-bonded ceramics for direct filling, or have indirect restoration such as inlays, onlays, crowns and veneers.

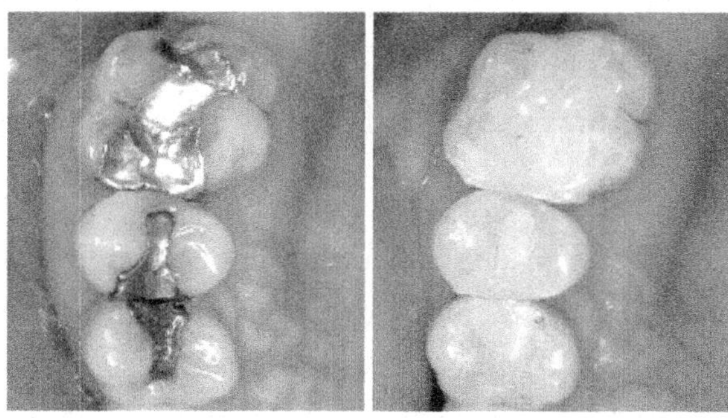

These images show the restoration of teeth before and after mercury fillings are removed

Special care must be taken when you're removing old mercury fillings to lessen your exposure to mercury toxins. One helpful step is to rinse your mouth first with a homeopathic mercury chelator (a binder of mercury). This is a great practice because the chelator coats the tissues so that it binds with mercury, and the heavy metal is easily washed away. It's applied twice; before the filling is removed, and then again right afterwards to capture any stray bits of mercury.

Before the filling is removed, a dental dam is applied to the inside of your mouth to help block particles of amalgam filling from contaminating you. A dental dam is a rubber-like fabric that has small holes placed in it that can be fitted over the teeth so that the teeth poke up through the material, thereby shielding the cheeks, gums and tongue away from the operating field. This technique of application is taught to all freshman year dental students but isn't widely used in practice. There are several types of dental dams available, and while none of them are 100 percent effective it does block a significant amount of particles from entering you. It's good to apply an additional layer of chelating cream to the dam to help further reduce your exposure to the mercury.

Dental dams give dentists a nice unobstructed view of the teeth we're working on, and a dry environment for placing the new filling material (direct resin). Moisture can contaminate the filling or the bond. If the slightest amount of moisture is present, even a breath, the almost invisible vapor that blankets the tooth will poison the bond and shorten the life of the filling. If the filling leaks and the tooth rots and you don't know it, the tooth could die, then abscess and cause you to be in a real pickle.

The main limitations for using a dental dam are a small mouth opening or wisdom teeth that get in the way. I urge my patients to give themselves the benefit of the doubt and try to have the dam placed. Almost always it can be placed with a bit of persistence, and the protection it offers is well worth it. Although not common, claustrophobic individuals don't do well with the dam. Then we work as rapidly as possible to rid the mouth of the particles.

A negative ion generator is another helpful device used during the removal of mercury fillings that assists in keeping the environment of the room where the treatment is taking place free of mercury ions. This tool creates a stream of charged ions from the "pitcher" that flows over your head and is collected by the "catcher." This treatment captures the mercury vapor that is created during the removal so the room and office environment is kept healthier.

To help remove any stray mercury particles in the air, we run a HEPA vacuum during the extraction. A HEPA filter has special agents held within a large canister that can trap multiple kinds of harmful and noxious materials. Mercury is but one of them. My assistant and I also wear masks approved by Occupational Safety & Health Administration (OSHA) and The National Institute for Occupational Safety and Health (NIOSH) that protect us from mercury vapor exposure.

We also use a nasal hood with positive pressure oxygen for our patients during the removal process because it creates a positive flow of oxygen into your nose, creating less of chance of you breathing in the mercury vapor.

Just prior to the application of the bonding agent or super glue that seals the tooth and adheres the filling, we use a different form of oxygen—ozone (O^3)—to sterilize the tooth and prepare the surface in the best possible way to receive the bonding agents. Our ozone is generated from medical grade oxygen. Not all dentists use ozone, but in my opinion, everyone would be well served if they did. It is fairly easy to dispense and is able to sterilize the tooth quickly. This helps to prevent future caries (decay).

Finally, I suggest an IV of Vitamin C. This helps neutralize the mercury that is mobilized from being locked in the tissues of your body via electrical balance. As your fillings are removed, there will be a redistribution of mercury and other heavy metals in your body as it attempts to rebalance with the new electrical balance that is dictated by a variety of factors. If you cannot have an IV, your next best option is to have an oral form of Vitamin C. Your doctor should be consulted for advice on the dose. Doing a detoxification can help bind the mercury in your body so your system can safely remove it through your elimination systems rather than reabsorbing it back into your tissues. There are organizations that can aid you in finding a physician near you that is capable of helping you with this aspect of your care.

You can go to www.DrNicholasMeyer.com to see all of my videos. To see a short video on ozone, go here:

For the safe removal of mercury fillings, go here:

The Problem with Metals

People often ask me if the other metals in their amalgam fillings, crowns and implants can also cause health problems. I tell them yes, and for a variety of reasons.

Common metals used in dentistry include copper, mercury, tin, zinc and silver. Amalgam fillings actually contain five different metals. Metal crowns can have two to five or more different metals. There are today over 500 different combinations of metals used in the creation of crowns and inlays in dentistry. Traditional partial dental frameworks have at least three metals: chrome, cobalt and molybdenum. But the trend is to move away from metals wherever possible.

One problem is that the metals dissociate or separate themselves in the presence of moisture and develop ions (charged metallic particles). These ions from the metals are constantly being released into your tissues (nerves, bone, blood, lymph) which can have a toxic effect on those cells.

Each person has a different sensitivity to these materials. One example of this phenomenon can be seen in the following images of an amalgam tattoo. The dark spots are made up of tiny metal particles from the filling or crown that become embedded in your tissue. They can appear on your gums, cheek, lips, tongue or the roof of your mouth.

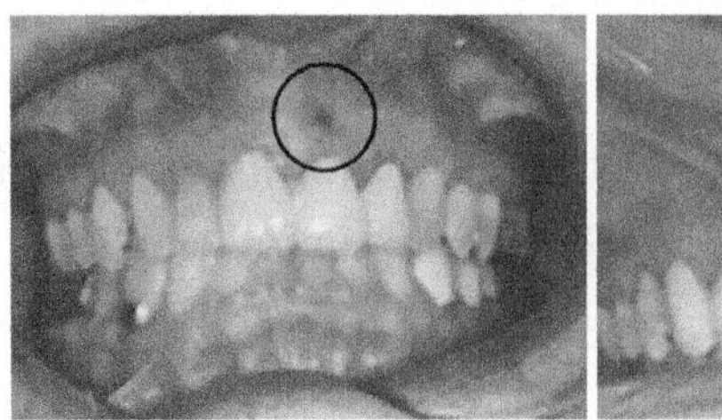
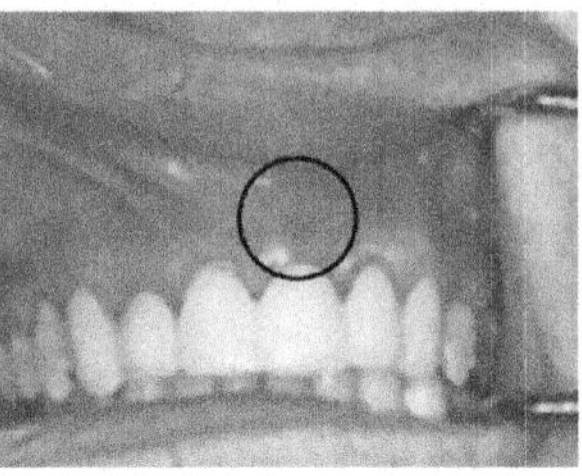

Before and after an amalgam tattoo was surgically removed

Another common problem with mercury fillings is that when your saliva contacts the metal of dental material, it thereby creates a measurable electrical current in your mouth. This is called oral galvanism.

One example of oral galvanism is when you bite on a piece of aluminum foil or touch your filling with a fork and it suddenly tastes metallic. Think of it as the metal boiling away from the surface of the filling. You can actually taste the metal that is being released.

This galvanism creates a measurable electric current that ranges from 20 millivolts to 200 or more millivolts in your mouth. Often it's greater than your body's usual 20 millivolts. I like to test the electro-galvanic activity of a patient's mouth during their dental examination.

Some people experience pain or other uncomfortable symptoms because of oral galvanism. You can also get headaches and skin irritations, like the amalgam tattoo shown above.[9]

For others, it's more difficult to understand or measure the effects of this constant electrical current on your body. It's similar to the way a woman doesn't look pregnant for several months, yet a baby is forming in all its complexity on its own set schedule. In much the same way, dental X-rays can't pick up that there's a cavity unless there's about 40 percent damage to the tooth. So a lot can go wrong below the surface before a problem is seen.

Galvanism has been found to affect your immune system, and it can cause symptoms like insomnia, vertigo and memory loss.[10] I see these kinds of symptoms regularly. Our brain is but inches away from the source of a lot of extraneous electrical activity (mixed metals), so it is impacted by this errant signaling that is considerably higher than the normal operational current of our body.

It is one reason people can have a seemingly miraculous recovery when their metal fillings are replaced, because there is an instantaneous removal of this electrical current that has been over-stimulating their system.

Safe Treatment

It is important to take precautions to safeguard your health. One thing I suggest is doing a Dental Materials Compatibility Test. It requires a fasting blood draw, centrifuging of the blood and then freezing it prior to overnight shipping.

This test compares your blood to scores of different dental materials, not just the fillings. You will get the results with an exhaustive listing of literally thousands of dental materials that are screened specifically for your safety and immune challenges. Things like bonding agents, impression materials, and the like. In general, the more health struggles you have, the more careful you need to be with your dental care and material selection. The last thing you want to do is throw gasoline onto a fire.

Since almost all dental materials have a biologic impact on the body, you have to take action to make sure you are using the safest materials for your long-term health. In today's world, nobody needs to be challenging their immune system unnecessarily. Everyone should realize that symptoms they are seeing might be due to the immune system effects of dental materials.

The goal is to eliminate or drastically reduce the "load" the body has to deal with that comes from dental treatments and the materials that are used to restore teeth. That's why I use materials that reduce oral galvanism and do not further challenge your immune system. I also use materials that are the least reactive with my patients' biochemistry according to their dental material compatibility testing.

Here are a few useful links to my website where you can see videos about mercury removal.

This video describes the preparations to have a mercury (amalgam) filling removed:

You may also wonder if insurance will cover your mercury filling removal? Go here to find out more:

How long should you wait in between mercury (amalgam) filling removals?

How many mercury (amalgam) fillings can I have removed at once?

Stainless Steel in the Mouth: The Dark Side of Shiny

Stainless steel is commonly used in orthodontics (tooth straightening) and in children's dentistry when they need to have a temporary crown for a tooth that will fall out or until they are older and a permanent crown can be placed. The problem with stainless steel is that it is an alloy of nickel and tin, and nickel is highly allergenic. Nickel is also used in the metal base of some dental bridges and under some porcelain crowns. It is strong, lightweight and relatively inexpensive compared to other metals such as gold and platinum.

There probably isn't a dentist alive (except newer graduates) who hasn't seen the side-effects from braces, usually the older style (train tracks), which can cause an overgrowth of gum tissue. While some dentists scold the child for not taking care of their teeth well enough, it often isn't their home care; it's their allergy to nickel that is wreaking havoc on their tissue.

As with most heavy metals, the problem doesn't stay in your mouth. Nickel sensitizes the immune system (think metalloproteins). When the immune system later encounters nickel, in jewelry for example or in body piercings, the body recognizes this and thus gives rise to negative effects in your body. Nickel can migrate elsewhere in your body, which causes you to become sensitized to the metal. A bigger reaction can occur later with additional exposure. An example of this is when people get their ears pierced and the posts cause a reaction because they are made out of nickel.

One of the more serious effects of nickel is that it lowers the lymphocyte levels (immune cells), and it can contribute to the development of cancer of the lungs, nose and larynx.[11]

I ask new patients if they have trouble wearing costume jewelry. If they answer yes then I know that they are metal sensitive and

I have to proceed with greater caution. Their immune system is already charged up or on alert and I want to be sure I can do all I can to not further compromise their health with the materials I use. I frequently advise them to take a Dental Materials Test. For ordering information, go to Chapter 12 – Holistic Dental Resources.

CASE STUDY

I was consulted by a concerned grandmother of a 5 year old girl. She felt that her granddaughter's behavior had changed after she had dental treatment and received four stainless steel crowns. The decision was made to change them out. Within a week or two the child's behavior returned to her previous normal self.

So What about Dental Implants?

Until recently in the U.S., only titanium or titanium alloy type dental implants were available for placement within the bone (intraosseous insertion). However European dentists pioneered the use of Zirconium Oxide implants, a ceramic type of material that is metal free. The FDA approved Zirconium Oxide for use in the U.S. in 2008. Now, as of this writing, we have a more versatile and user-friendly two-piece Zirconium Oxide dental implant available, which is a very good thing.

Dental implants are important because you need a proper bite platform in order to create the right amount of force while you're chewing. That helps maintain your well-being because the resistance of our teeth against each other (or against a dental implant) keeps our muscles functioning soundly and prevents TMD problems (see Chapter 4 – TMD and Airway Disorders: I Haven't Got Time for the Pain).

Furthermore, a dental implant means you won't necessarily need to get dentures or a removable prosthetic device. That can make all the difference in having clearer pronunciation, appearance and function. There is an interesting relationship between the amount of space in your mouth and airway, and the amount of air that you can pass through to your lungs. Small changes (either an increase or decrease) can have a big effect in the volume of air that can pass through.

Not only that, the bone in your jaw tends to deteriorate over time without teeth in place. Dental implants give the bone purpose again and your jaw bone can be preserved from certain demise.

There is not universal agreement within the holistic community on the use of dental implants. My view is that whatever is done for someone is a compromise from the wholeness of the teeth. Our efforts are aimed at helping restore as optimum function as possible to an individual, bearing in mind the overall health status and potential troubles that may occur in the future.

Health Effects

Allergies are the most common problem caused by the metal in dental implants. Unless you test for materials compatibility, you won't know if your implants are causing the problem. Science backs up this theory, with a number of articles written in the medical literature about allergies to medical and dental implants.[12]

Many of the older problems with dental implants have been solved, but a question that commonly comes up is whether there's enough bone left to do an implant. This can be determined by a 3D CT dental scan or cone beam, which gives off a lot lower radiation than its medical counterpart. Since you have to have bone for an implant, it's not uncommon for bone grafting to be recommended. That will help ensure a more successful outcome.

Another issue that can occur is when the implant doesn't match your other teeth positionally. That can be a limitation of the straight single-piece zirconium oxide implant versus the newer two piece implant. The new implants are snow white and much more color compatible than the older metal implants.

Safe Treatment

If titanium implants are causing health issues, they may be replaced with zirconium oxide implants. That's what I recommend, as do others who practice holistic dentistry. Zirconia, the metal, can pass electrons, while zirconium oxide can't pass electrons therefore it is no longer considered to be a metal. So it doesn't cause the same harmful effects, like oral galvanism.

That means there is a vastly reduced risk of allergy or sensitivity issues. At the same time, these ceramic implants provide the positive benefits of titanium implants by preventing the deterioration of bone in the jaw that can occur over time.

The zirconium oxide implants have other benefits as well. They are durable and don't easily corrode from the acids in your saliva and food. They're also less temperature sensitive. Food can be chewed normally, because the tooth or teeth generally feels and functions the same as natural teeth. The implant has a natural look and it blends well with the rest of the teeth in the mouth. It's the more natural solution to the problem of titanium allergy.

Conclusion

This chapter is meant to make you aware of this simple fact: what you put into your body dictates your health and well-being. Unfortunately, there have been so many special interests intervening in your health for the sake of profit that it's difficult to sort through the morass. I hope this information will help you make a more informed choice when it comes to the dental materials you put in your body.

End Notes

[1] "EPA Memorandum of Understanding on Reducing Dental Amalgam Discharges." *Dental Effluent Guidelines*. Environmental Protection Agency. Web. 25 Feb. 2016.

[2] Legal brief filed in 1995 by attorneys for the ADA in W.H. Tolhurst vs. Johnson and Johnson Consumer Products, Inc.; Engelhard Corporation; ABE Dental, Inc.; the American Dental Association, et al., in the Superior

Court of the State of California, in and for the County of Santa Clara, CA, Case No. 718228.

[3] U.S. Patent 4,018,600 (April, 1977): https://www.google.com/patents/US4018600?dq=4,018,600&hl=en&sa=X&ei=KEuIVbHdO8-eoQSa0baoBA&ved=0CB0Q6AEwAA U.S. Patent 4,078,921 (March, 1978): https://www.google.com/patents/US4078921?dq=4,078,921&hl=en& sa=X&ei=Z0uIVfvbD5XroATOi4sQ&ved=0CB4Q6AEwAA

[4] "Dental Amalgam, Mercury, and Amalgam Alloy." *Class II Special Controls Guidance Document.* U.S. Food and Drug Administration. Web. 25 Feb. 2016.

[5] "Lawsuit Filed Today Against FDA for Failing to Address Risks of Mercury in Dental Fillings - IAOMT." *IAOMT.* International Academy of Oral Medicine and Toxicology, 05 Mar. 2014. Web. 25 Feb. 2016.

[6] Queen, H.L. "Chronic Mercury Toxicity: New Hope Against an Endemic Disease." (1988) Web. 25 Feb. 2016.

[7] University of Calgary Medical School. "Brain Neuron Degeneration via Mercury." (September 17, 2006). Web. 25 Feb. 2016: https://www.youtube.com/watch?v=IHqVDMr9ivo&list=PLKXWn2R77hJCKt8thiXIj-8ID-dFKja1X

[8] Vimy, M.J., N.D. Boyd, D.E. Hooper, and F.L. Lorscheider. "Glomerular filtration impairment by mercury released from dental 'silver' fillings in sheep." *The Physiologist* (August 15, 1990).

[9] Kucerová, H., T. Dostálová, J. Procházková, J. Bártová, and L. Himmlová. "Influence of galvanic phenomena on the occurrence of algic symptoms in the mouth." *Gen Dent.* 50.1 (2002): 62-65.

[10] Podzimek, S., M. Tomka, P. Sommerova, Y. Lyuya-Mi, J. Bartova, and J. Prochazkova. "Immune markers in oral discomfort patients before and

after elimination of oral galvanism." *Neuro Endocrinol Lett.* 34.8 (2013): 802-808.

[11] Eggleston, D. "Effect of Dental Amalgam and Nickel Alloys on T-Lymphocytes: Preliminary Report." *Journal of Prosthetic Dent.* 51.5 (1984): 617-623.

[12] Javed, F., K. Al-Hezaimi, and G.E. Romanos. "Is titanium sensitivity associated with allergic reactions in patients with dental implants? A systematic review." *Clin Implant Dent Relat Res.* 15.1 (February, 2013): 47-52.

CHAPTER 3

FLUORIDE: MORE FOE THAN FRIEND?

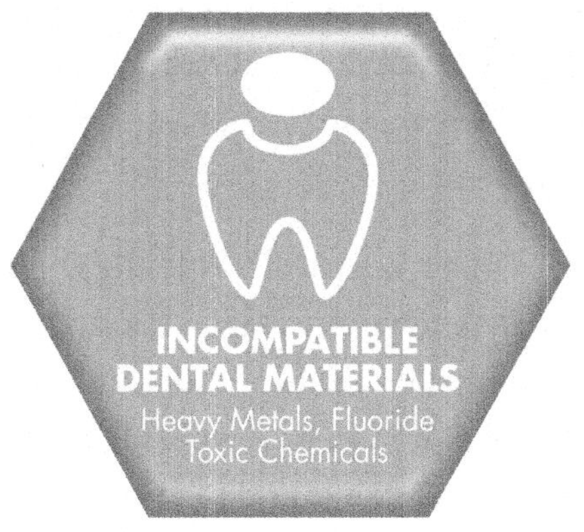

Fluoride is now everywhere. You almost can't get away from it in the United States. The widespread practice of dosing the public with fluoride in the water was first approved by the government in 1945 as a study sponsored by the Surgeon General to prove that fluoridation would prevent cavities in children.

After a decade of adding fluoride to the local water supply in Grand Rapids, Michigan, the project (which was taken up by the National Institute of Dental Research) found tooth decay dropped more than 60 percent among almost 30,000 schoolchildren.[1]

Since then, water fluoridation has been heralded as one of the ten great public health achievements of the 20th century by the Centers for Disease Control and Prevention. The current claim by the CDC is that water fluoridation reduces tooth decay by 25 percent.[2]

Yet even though fluoride is used for cavity prevention, tooth decay is not actually a fluoride deficiency—as scurvy is a Vitamin C deficiency. The fluoride that is added to water and toothpaste is intended to harden the enamel of your teeth to make them more resistant to decay.

Unfortunately that's not all fluoride does. Fluoride upsets a protein in our body known as collagen, causing damage to bones, teeth, connective tissue, arteries and skin. Basically fluoride unwraps the collagen protein molecule, making it unsuitable for its intended purpose in all of our body tissues.

It took the powerful commercial interests of industry and healthcare to conspire to force you to be medicated through our water system. In particular there were the political efforts led by the U.S. Public Health Service and the American Dental Association that brought about the practice of public water fluoridation.

If you have symptoms of irritability, anxiety, nervousness with difficulty breathing, you may be suffering from fluoride exposure. It can also cause abdominal cramps, diarrhea or constipation. It can even cause stiffness and lack of mobility.

Check out the Holistic Dental Matrix to see the full list of symptoms that can be caused by fluoride.

How Did Our Water Get Fluoridated?

You probably don't know that the fluoride in our water started out as an industrial waste byproduct. Yes, that's right. Fluoride is a waste product of aluminum production. For the first half of the twentieth century, manufacturers just dumped the fluoride wherever they could, like rivers and landfills. But it was discovered that the fluoride was poisoning nearby crops and making livestock sick.

For the Aluminum Company of America (ALCOA), the largest producer of fluoride waste, this was a problem. When the link between fluoride and tooth decay was discovered independently by several researchers in 1931, ALCOA founder Andrew Mellon arranged for Public Health Service dentist, Henry Trendley Dean, to go study remote towns in the Western U.S. where water wells have a naturally high concentration of calcium fluorides. Henry Trendley Dean helped to identify a causal link between high concentrations of fluoride in the drinking water and mottled tooth enamel through epidemiological studies. He created a classification system for dental fluorosis that is still used today called Dean's Index.[3]

The Mellon Institute was started by Andrew Mellon, owner of ALCOA, specifically in order to produce research that supported industry. For example, for several decades the Mellon Institute produced research showing that asbestos was safe and did not cause cancer. This kind of research was intended to help companies who were trying to find ways to get rid of their toxic waste products, such as the Aluminum Company of America (ALCOA), the Aluminum Company of Canada, American Petroleum Institute, DuPont, Kaiser Aluminum, Reynolds Steel and US Steel.

In 1939, one of the Mellon Institute scientists Gerald J. Cox, stated, "The present trend toward removal of fluorides from food and water may need reversal," and he contended that a maximum allowable fluoride contaminant level of 1 part per million (ppm) would prevent dental cavities. The Mellon Institute also produced reports supported by the American Dental Association that assured everyone that fluoride was not toxic and would be beneficial to add to our drinking water for healthy teeth.

The Pentagon Scientific Research and Development Group further pursued the project to fluoridate the drinking water, and their members included Henry L. Barnett, a captain in the Manhattan Project medical section, along with John W. Fertig, SRDG, Dr. Hodge, and David Ast, chief dental officer of the New York State Health Department, who was placed in charge of the Newburg Project. From 1944 to 1948, the group was looking for information on the cumulative effects of fluoride.

Previously classified documents from Manhattan Project included numerous studies that found fluoride was detrimental to living organisms. An April 29, 1944 Manhattan Project memo, released in 1997, states: "Clinical evidence suggests that uranium hexafluoride may have a rather marked central nervous system effect, with mental confusion, drowsiness and lassitude as the conspicuous features... it seems that the fluoride component is the causative factor....since work with these compounds is essential, it will be necessary to know in advance what mental effects may occur after exposure, if workmen are to be properly protected. This is important not only to protect a given individual, but also to prevent a confused workman from injuring others by improperly performing his duties."[4]

Indeed, in 1950, the 24th edition of the U.S. Dispensatory defined fluorides as "violent poisons to all living tissue because of their precipitation of calcium. They cause fall of blood pressure, respiratory failure, and general paralysis. Continuous ingestion of non-fatal doses causes permanent inhibition of growth ... the use of fluoride-containing dentifrices and internal medicaments is not justified."[5]

Yet at the same time, the U.S. Public Health Service officially endorsed the concept of adding fluorides to public water supplies. Coincidentally, that was the same year that the ALCOA Aluminum's Vancouver, Washington plant was found guilty of dumping 7,000 pounds of toxic fluorides each month into the Columbia River. According to the *Seattle Times*, "the fluoride contaminated the grass and forage and resulted in injury and death to cattle."[6]

In subsequent editions of the U.S. Dispensatory, the editors removed the section about fluoride because it became politically correct to support ongoing public fluoridation programs in order to prevent tooth decay. Propaganda campaigns also helped encourage the public use of fluoride to prevent cavities.

Dr. John Yiamouyiannis discusses this intrigue in his book *Fluoride: The Aging Factor*, in which the early days of fluoridation read like a fast-paced thriller filled with subterfuge and financial payoffs. George Orwell in his book *1984* couldn't have been more accurate about what played out behind closed doors when it comes to fluoride.

With a Ph.D. in biochemistry, Yiamouyiannis cites numerous references for studies that confirmed the risks of fluoridation well before the 1990s. His book is called *Fluoride: The Aging Factor* because that's what fluoride does. It ages us prematurely, from the moment we take our first contaminated drink.

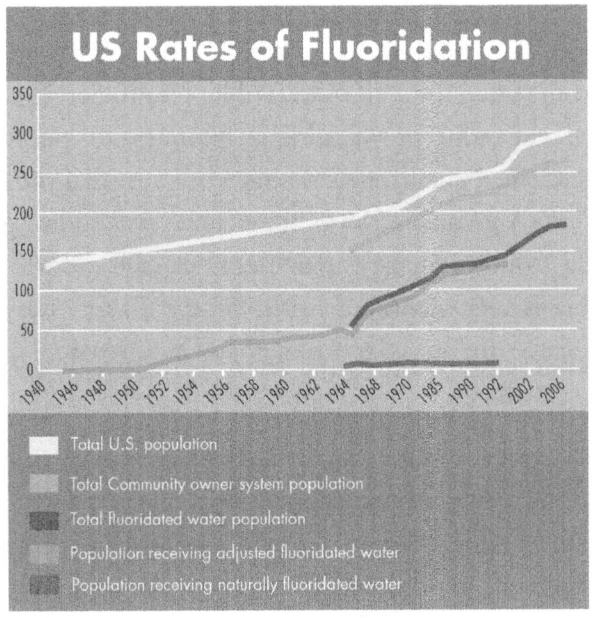

The rate of exposure to fluoride has risen sharply according to the CDC

Fluoride Exposure

Ironically today, it is illegal to dump fluoride into our lakes and rivers, but it is perfectly fine to put in our drinking water and toothpaste. Gee, this sounds very similar to the mercury in our mouths! And since commercial crops are watered with fluoridated water, they absorb the fluoride. Fruit juices from concentrate are reconstituted with fluoridated water, and bottled water often has fluoride in it.

Nearly 75 percent of U.S. citizens who are served by public water systems receive fluoridated water. If you're wondering about your own public water, the CDC has a handy chart of all the public water systems and whether they are fluoridated: https://nccd.cdc.gov/DOH_MWF/Default/Default.aspx

But the CDC chart won't tell you what other kinds of chemicals are being added to your water. To find out, you have to ask your local supplier for their water report.

Originally sodium fluoride was used to fluoridate public drinking water, but now less than 10 percent of water systems nationwide use this form. Today the main fluoride chemical added to water is hydrofluorosilicic acid, which is an industrial by-product from the phosphate fertilizer industry. It is consumed by over 140 million people in the U.S.

Silicofluorides are unlicensed medicinal substances that have never been submitted to the FDA for approval. They are banned in most of Europe, and the European Union human rights legislation makes it illegal to fluoridate the water with them.[7]

In 1999, Dartmouth researchers found high levels of lead in children who drink silicofluorides, which has been confirmed by additional studies.[8]

Plenty of scientists have spoken out against the modern-day use of fluoride in our water. Dr. William Marcus, Senior Science Advisor to the EPA Office of Water, was fired because of his outspoken opposition to water fluoridation in the early 1990s. The U.S. Secretary of Labor, Robert Reich, later ruled that EPA fired Marcus out of "retaliation" for Marcus' stance on fluoride, and ordered EPA to reinstate Marcus with full back pay and compensation.[9]

Similarly, researcher Dr. Phyllis Mullenix was asked to study fluoride, and she was surprised to find that fluoride is a neurotoxin and causes effects like hyperactivity, memory problems, and IQ problems similar to ADD/ADHD in laboratory rats.[10] After submitting her findings, she was fired from the Harvard-affiliated Forsyth Dental Research Center and her career as a grant-funded research scientist was destroyed.

It wasn't until April, 2015, in response to the growing body of scientific studies that have found that over-exposure to fluoride contributes to serious health concerns, that the U.S. Health and Human Services (HHS) finally lowered the recommended level of fluoride to 0.7 milligrams per liter of water. This replaces the previous recommended range (0.7 to 1.2 milligrams per liter) issued in 1962.[11] Yet the EPA still has not yet come out with any revised Maximum Contaminant Levels for fluoride, so water suppliers don't have to conform to the HHS recommendations.

Health Effects

We know fluoride is bad for your body. There's no system that is not disrupted by the presence of the fluoride ion (Fl^-): it damages enzymes and proteins, upsets our immune system, and can cause autoimmune diseases. It even damages our DNA, which can cause tumors and cancer. Fluoride builds up in your body over a lifetime, much like heavy metals do. So the serious problems usually begin to show up in middle age.

One of the earliest and most readily visible effects of fluoride on the body is called "dental fluorosis." That's when your teeth get a mottled appearance. It can be as mild as small blotches on the teeth or as severe as teeth that are brown and heavily pitted. I see mottling every day in my office. It's an epidemic.

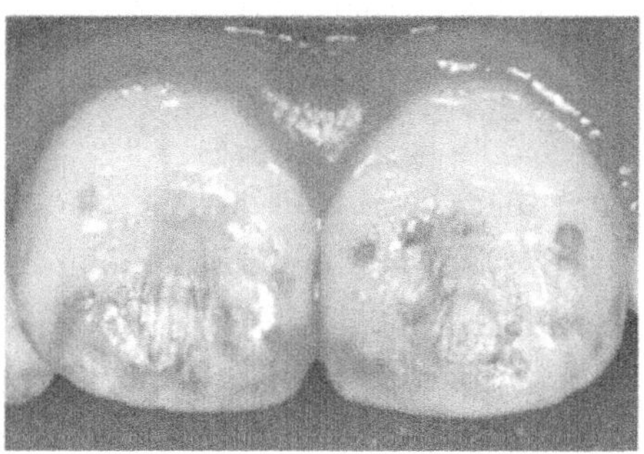

Moderate mottling of teeth caused by fluoride exposure

However it's the things we can't see that can be more of a problem. The same process of fluorosis hardens not only the crystal structure of teeth but also bone. So when you are older, particularly if you're a woman, you are at a much higher risk of hip fractures because of the additional fluoride in your system.

There are also unfortunately cases of childhood death after fluoride poisoning. If you read the label of any brand of toothpaste that contains fluoride you will see a warning that if a child swallows more than a *pea* sized amount of the tooth paste, you're to take them immediately to the poison control center.

Yet how is toothpaste sold in commercials? With the whole brush full of paste and a cute little upturn on the end, often with star. The message is obvious: put a whole wad of toothpaste on your brush to get maximum exposure to the great ingredients.

One of the biggest problems with fluoride over-exposure is that it hurts your thyroid gland. Your thyroid sits at the base of your neck and helps regulate the other glands in your system. We cannot live without it. Yet our thyroid can appear to be working well, and blood tests will confirm it, even when it's not. That's because the fluoride ion (F-) competes with iodine for binding sites within the thyroid gland (the hormones T3 and T4).[12]

So your doctor may think your thyroid gland is fine because your T3 and T4 blood tests show functioning levels, but really there's an imposter present. Sort of like a movie plot where an evil twin sabotages the good twin's life, while the good twin doesn't realize there's a problem. You could have hypothyroidism without it showing up on the tests, while you're complaining about symptoms of lethargy, weight gain and always feeling cold.

Are you getting the picture? You can have a normal blood test even though you're not feeling good, all because fluoride can mask a nonfunctioning thyroid. This problem can be even worse when we add in mercury to the mix, which can result in Hashimoto's thyroiditis, an autoimmune disorder. Even though your thyroid is ready and willing to work, it can't fulfill its mission because it has been poisoned. If you think this might be your problem, it's wise to see a knowledgeable doctor who is familiar with basal temperature diagnosis and use of natural thyroid supplements.

Safe Treatment

Holistic dentistry advises that you use non-fluoridated polishing pastes and no fluoride rinses. This is especially true for children who can't tolerate high levels of fluoride. If fluoride is a real problem for you, there are fluoride eliminating systems for your home that can cut down on your exposure.

At the very least, reduce your exposure to fluoride. Drink water that hasn't been fluoridated—check the labels on bottled water to be sure you're not getting fluoride that way. Many bottled waters today have up to 1.4 mg of fluoride per liter, which is twice the level of the new recommended guidelines. You *must* read the labels. Package designers are clever and there are a goodly number of "natural" toothpastes that contain fluoride.

One of the popular sayings out there now is that drinking fluoride to protect the outer layer of your teeth is like drinking sunscreen to protect your skin. There are better ways to prevent decay by using a topical, natural solution rather than ingesting fluoride. Some natural alternatives for fluoride toothpaste are brushing with sea salt, baking soda or hydrogen peroxide. Essential oils, coconut oil, or herbal tooth powders can also be used for cleaning. Some people prefer to brush with plain water or use a Waterpic® for oral irrigation.

If you have been diagnosed with hypothyroidism, you should discuss your treatment with your doctor and include your concerns about fluoride treatments, fluoride toothpaste and water consumption (including bottled). You have to take into account that the dose is cumulative. Your dentist can help by not throwing fuel onto the fire. By that I mean not prescribing additional fluoride use for home, or using fluoride products in the office.

Other Dental Material Issues

A seldom-heard-of illness termed Neurocutaneous Syndrome (NCS) was first identified in the literature in 2004 as being related to dental toxicity, according to Dr. Omar M. Amin, PhD.[13] This disorder is characterized by certain skin eruptions which have the appearance of Morgellons Disease. The jury is still out on that but it does not seem to be related. NCS is characterized by "weeping sores" that appear on the face, neck, trunk and other places. It is believed to be brought on by exposure to dental materials.

Often in attempting to draw a connection from the insult to the manifestation there is a time lag. The lag is usually not on the short side of life. Thus, one usually will not connect a dental event to the skin eruptions. Furthermore, even if the patient suspects that there is a connection, if a dentist is quizzed about it they would most likely say, "No, dental materials don't create that type of reaction."

According to Amin, one of the chemicals that causes NCS is ethyltoluene sulfonamide. This product can be found in filling liners—ask your dentist if it's in the product he uses. Dentists are obligated to provide the MSDS of the materials being used upon request.

Ethyltoluene sulfonamide may be a mouthful, but broken down we find the first part, ethyltoluene is a neurotoxin (poison to the brain) and was reported to be used by the Nazi's during World War II as one of their chemical weapons. The other half of the term is sulfonamide. This part of the compound is a sulfur compound. Experience has revealed that a large swath of the population is sensitive to the sulfur class of antibiotics and must watch out for them like a hawk.

So here you are with a cavity and the doctor is about to restore the tooth with the filling and they innocently place this liner material into the cavity preparation prior to the insertion of the filling. So now you have a toxic substance in your body.

When this substance is placed on your freshly exposed tooth structure, which is porous, it will be carried through your body by way of the blood stream. The filling is out of sight and out of mind and seldom, if ever, considered to be a source of the toxin that is setting off the reaction.

The list of suspects can be overwhelming. Thankfully, for the most part, it seems that the body deals well with the toxins that are held in the materials used within the oral cavity.

Conclusion

The holistic dentistry approach contributes to your overall health in a way that traditional dentistry does not in regard to the choice and use of dental materials that are safe for your immune system. That's why holistic dentistry can restore your teeth and enhance your health and well-being. If you don't pay attention to these basic principles, all kinds of illness can manifest, sometimes years down the line.

End Notes

[1] Murthy, V.H. "Community Water Fluoridation: One of CDC's "10 Great Public Health Achievements Of The 20th Century." *Public Health Reports* 130 (2015).

[2] "Community Water Fluoridation." *Centers for Disease Control and Prevention*. Centers for Disease Control and Prevention, 2015. Web. 24 Feb. 2016.

[3] Fejerskov O., and E.A.M. Kidd. *Dental Caries: The Disease and Its Clinical Management.* John Wiley & Sons, 2009: 299–327.

[4] Previously classified SECRET Manhattan Project Memo, April 29, 1944, declassified and released from the National Archives. Retrieved February 25, 2016, from http://qbit.cc/blog/wp-content/uploads/2011/04/FLUORIDE_-_Fluoridation_Chronology__V._Good_1.pdf

[5] Osol, A., and G.E. Farrar. *The Dispensatory of the United States of America* [The 24th Edition]. J. B. Lippincott Company, 1947: 1456-1457.

[6] Reported by the *Seattle Times*, Dec. 15, 1952.

[7] Cross, D.W., and R.J. Carton R.J. "Fluoridation: a violation of medical ethics and human rights." *Int J Occup Environ Health* 9.1 (Jan-Mar 2003): 24-9.

[8] Coplan, M.J., S.C. Patch, R.D. Masters, and M.S. Bachman. "Confirmation of and explanations for elevated blood lead and other disorders in children exposed to water disinfection and fluoridation chemicals." *Neurotoxicology* 28.5 (2005): 1032-42.

[9] "Scientist Who Spoke Out on Fluoride Ordered Reinstated to Job." *The Associated Press* Feb. 11, 1994.

[10] Mullenix, P.J., P.K. Denbesten, A. Schunior, and W.J. Kernan. "Neurotoxicity of sodium fluoride in rats." *Neurotoxicology and Teratology* 17.2 (March–April 1995): 169–177.

[11] U.S. Department of Health & Human Services. "HHS issues final recommendation for community water fluoridation." Retrieved February 25, 2016 from http://www.hhs.gov/news/press/2015pres/04/20150427a.html

[12] Chandna, S. and M. Bathla. "Oral manifestations of thyroid disorders and its management." *Indian J Endocrinol Metab* 15.Suppl2 (July 2011): S113–S116.

[13] Amin, O.M. "Dental Sealant Toxicity: Neurocutaneous Syndrome (NCS), a dermatological and neurological disorder." *Holistic Dental Association Journal: The Communicator* 1 (2004): 1-15.

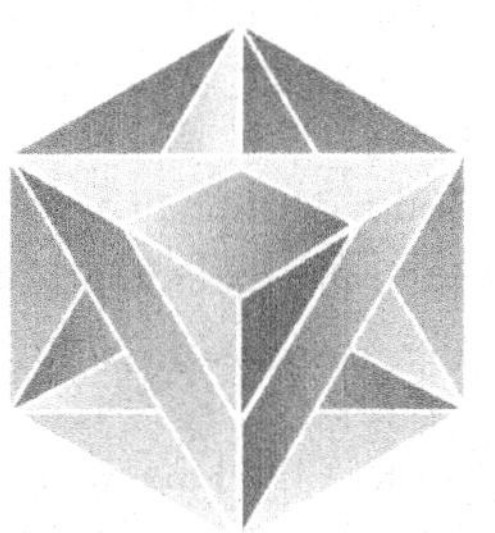

CHAPTER 4

TMD AND AIRWAY DISORDERS: I HAVEN'T GOT TIME FOR THE PAIN

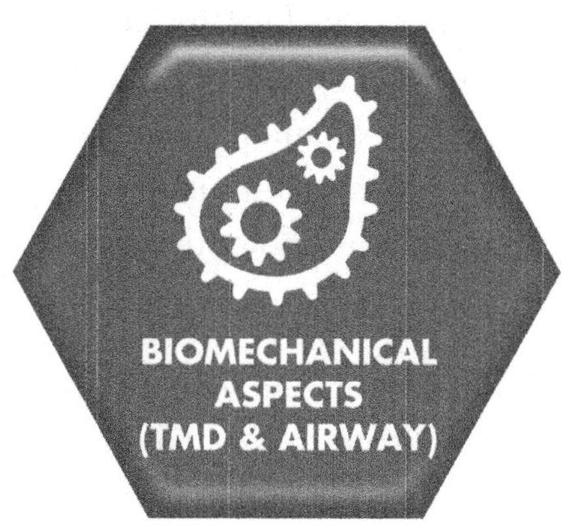

If you found your symptoms in my Holistic Dental Matrix™ and you were sent to this chapter, then the root of your problem may be a Temporomandibular Joint Disorder (TMD) or an airway disorder or both. Not only are many head and neck problems caused by TMD and airway disorders, but a bad bite can also affect your heart, your gastrointestinal tract, systemic issues and even behavioral conditions.

There are 50 documented symptoms alone in my Holistic Dental Matrix that can be related to TMD problems. The myriad of presentations is so well-known that this condition has been referred to as "The Great Imposter." That's because you may have no way of knowing your symptoms are coming from a misaligned, overworked bite or other factors.

You may not even have pain in your jaw and yet you're suffering in other parts of your body. In fact, when you compare your symptoms to what you see in the Holistic Dental Matrix with those of fibromyalgia, mold allergy, sensitivity, hypothyroidism or Lyme disease, you will often find the same joint pains, muscle pains, sleep disturbances, headaches, difficulty concentrating, numb sensations in the extremities, brain fog, etc. I'm mostly talking about the biomechanical (motions of the parts and how they interact) aspects of your body that you've probably never thought about before.

I have to admit, it's quite an amazing thing. One answer lies in your nervous system, that wonderful part of your body that keeps us "wired and alive." Our nervous system is designed to coordinate our motions and emotions, both voluntary and involuntary, by transmitting signals from one part of our body to another. That communication sets up a chain reaction.

Healthy communication within your body depends on:

Nutrition – the foods we eat and don't eat

Neurology – how our brain processes the information

Endocrinology – how hormones regulate our body responses

Stress – how we process chemicals caused by stress

Your body is designed for harmony and balance amongst the various parts—*all of them!* When there's an imbalance, that's when dysfunction and breakdown takes place somewhere else in your body.

The problem is that modern medicine is geared to specialization, with more doctors treating certain parts of your body instead of looking at you as a whole. Is it any wonder our healthcare costs are sky high?

CASE STUDY

Several months ago, a 70-year-old female patient of mine went to the emergency room one night for chest pains. She was admitted for three days and a series of tests were run. All of the results were normal.

Her attending cardiologist informed her that nothing was amiss and that she was to be released that day. She told the doctor, "But, Doctor, I'm so tired." To which he replied, "There's nothing wrong and it's time to go." While her daughter gathered her things, my patient sat down in a chair still attached to her monitors. Right there she suffered a heart attack! Sitting still in her room after being told, "There's nothing wrong with you."

You may be in the same position—doctors have told you there's nothing wrong with you, and that your tests came out normal. Yet you feel bad.

So let's look deeper and see if the root of your problems comes from a faulty bite.

TMD Disorders

The reason I've put TMD and airway disorders together in this chapter is because they involve the same physical structures of the nose, throat, mouth and jaws. These are very complex, moving structures made up of bones, muscles, teeth, organs (your tongue) and the connective tissue that hold all of the parts together with nerves carrying the action/feedback signals. It is like watching a symphony in motion.

The airway passages (hollow spaces) are lined by soft tissue, for the most part, and the TMD tissues are considered both the harder tissues and soft tissues. Many doctors consider airway issues to be like the reverse side of the coin of TMD issues, yet we need to honor and treat each disorder differently depending on the nature of the disturbance and location of the tissues involved. With this integrated viewpoint, I think you will agree they are inseparable.

You may have also heard of TM disorders referred to as TMJ, the term in common usage for Temporomandibular Disorders.[1] The temporomandibular joint connects your lower jaw bone to the temporal bone of your skull in front of your ear. You have matching joints on either side of your face that serve as a hinge for your jaw.

Multiple muscles power this joint, and there's a tiny disc, the size of a nickel in the shape of a donut, composed of cartilage positioned between the two bones. It's said to be the most-used joint in the body. When you talk, chew, kiss, swallow and breathe, you're using this joint.

There is also a band of soft tissue that lives in the back part of the joint. It is highly elastic and is responsible for pulling the little disc back into position when you close your mouth. For many reasons, this tissue can be fairly easily injured and can be responsible for the pains you experience.

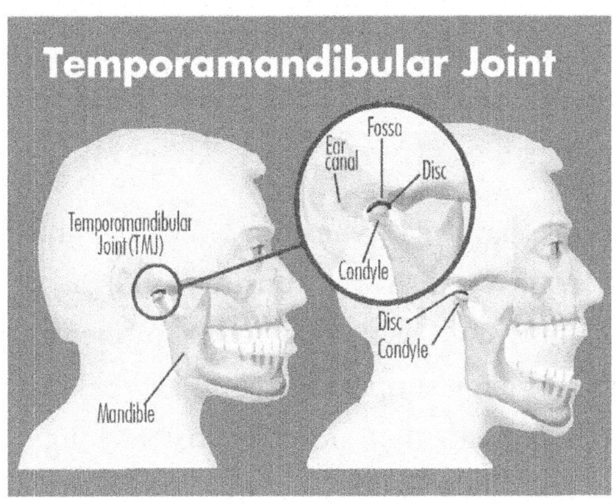

This is the temporomandibular joint

I've also included Myofascial Pain Syndrome in TMD disorders, which is muscle pain caused by inflammation in your body's soft tissues. There is also Craniomandibular Dysfunction, which is a group of disorders caused by damage to the nerves and muscles of the jaw joints and several other related structures of the mouth and throat.

A TMD problem often, but not always, occurs when your jaw joints don't function smoothly and harmoniously. Since so many systems are involved—teeth, bones, muscles and nervous system—a problem in any of these areas can have much wider repercussions for your health. TMD issues can even arise when there are well functioning jaw joints, too.

There are many reasons why your chewing muscles and jaw joints may not work together properly. A bite can malfunction because of: natural growth and development that goes awry; accidents and falls; lack of dental care or improper/inadequate care; compressive overload from clenching or grinding; and even emotions that cause you to clench and/or grind your jaw. These are all forms of stress.

Some people have malocclusion, which is a misalignment or incorrect relation between the teeth and the jaws. That means your upper and lower teeth don't meet properly, so you don't have the right bracing support for your jaw. This can come from missing teeth or teeth that are too short or long. Or differing-sized upper and lower jaws, or a mismatch between your jaw size and shape compared to your tooth size. Any one of these things can cause tooth overcrowding and abnormal bite patterns. However, just because you have this doesn't automatically mean you will develop a TMD problem.

The most common reason for bite malfunction is trauma. It could be macro type trauma, for example the kind you get when you're in a car accident, or the micro trauma that comes from grinding or clenching your teeth (they are related but different). Many people engage in we call a "parafunctional habit" like tooth grinding, tongue-thrusting, fingernail biting and pen chewing which are different forms of trauma.

In particular, tooth grinding (or gnashing) is an epidemic. I've seen the number of patients who are suffering from this escalate in recent years, and the age range of those who do it is getting lower. Grinding is when you unconsciously move your jaws with your teeth together either during the daytime or while sleeping (sleep bruxism).

Health Effects

So there you are: your teeth and gums are melting away before your eyes because of a bad habit, but you're thinking you have no hormones because of menopause and your doctor and your research on the Internet says that having no estrogen causes gum loss. But I can tell you in no uncertain terms, you have likely been grossly misinformed and uninformed by a well-intentioned person in a white coat who doesn't know beans about the functional maladies of teeth. To properly diagnose your condition takes more than a faceless array of digital diagnostic tools. You need the knowledge to interpret what you're seeing.

Too many people end up on a medical merry-go-round that only looks at your individual symptoms as the primary trouble when the diagnosis is really TMD. That leads to frustration, wasted time, and potentially to an exhausted bank account.

That's why I developed my Holistic Dental Matrix as a kind of secret decoder ring, to help you figure out what is really going wrong. Holistic dentistry can help you diagnose the real problem when symptoms are appearing in different areas of your body. That's because holistic dentistry looks at you as a whole. I often see problems associated directly with teeth since I'm a dentist, but long ago I realized that more often than not, more is going on than the tooth that presents itself as the problem.

TMD is often a progressive disorder resulting in significant alteration of the "ball" of your jaw joint if it is allowed to continue without intervention. When your jaw isn't in alignment as it moves, it can cause a series of compression injuries. Typically when this happens, the disc of cartilage that sits between the bones of your skull and lower jaw slips forward. This is what is responsible for the clicking or popping you may experience. Without the cartilage between the bones, they rub against each other and press directly on the nerve endings.

You may also feel clicking or popping with TMD. The pressure can be great enough that the cartilage deteriorates and sounds gravely when you open and close your mouth.

Once your jaw joints are displaced, that can cause muscle spasms that can stimulate your nerves, causing pain in or around the jaw. The pain can spread to your neck and shoulders, or into your head in the form of a muscle contraction headache caused by the repetition of clenching your jaw muscles. The muscle spasms can also cause lockjaw, which is a limited opening of your mouth.

Not only that, but unhealthy nerve signals are generated as your teeth are contacting each other when they grind. Those signals travel to your brain through your Trigeminal Nerve, also called Cranial Nerve 5. This nerve is the largest and most complex of the cranial nerves—it's the big boy on the block. It takes part in processing the signals that go through the limbic system of your brain.

The limbic system is your primitive reptilian brain. It's responsible for the emotional part of our lives, and it triggers the fight or flight reaction in our nervous system.

So just think, if you grind your teeth at night, you are keeping your nervous system working in high gear for hours every night. Your adrenal glands are pumping out the stress hormone cortisol in response, so you develop adrenal fatigue and you get moody. Physical stress also triggers constant muscle activity and can cause muscle overload and pain all over your body.

Then, to make matters worse, you can become addicted or habituated to the stress, and you begin to carry the habit of grinding your teeth from nighttime into daytime.

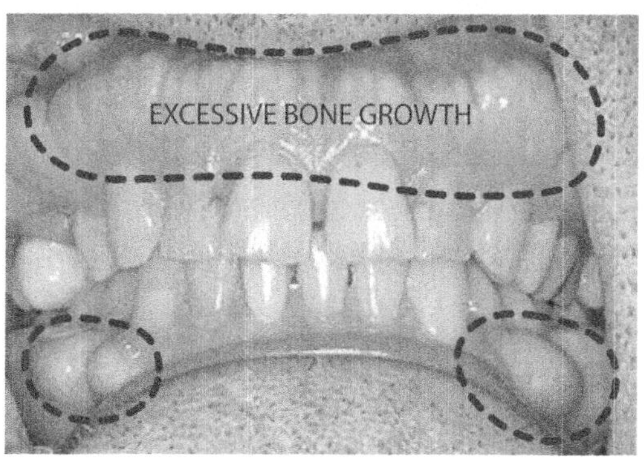

Physical stress can cause this type of bone distortion

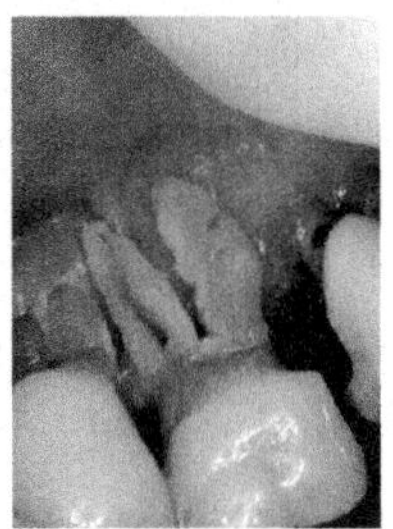

Exposed root

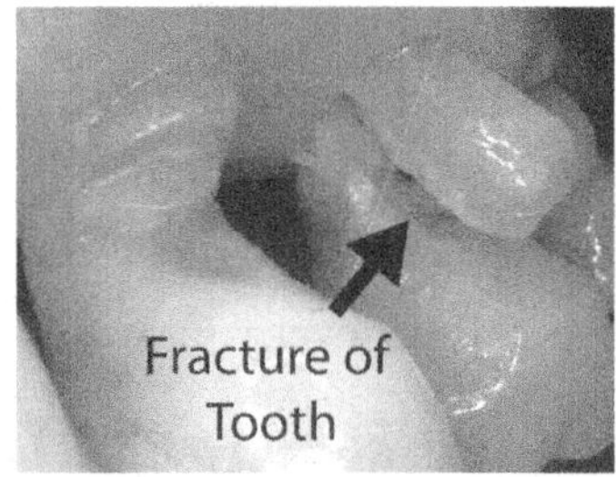

Physical stress also causes this painless tooth destruction

Cranial Nerve 5 is also the root cause of migraines for some people. Though the exact relationship is not known, during "migraine attacks" as your trigeminal nerve signals for the release of neuropeptides, researchers have found that serotonin levels drop, which is what causes the pain.[2] One thing is certain: if you tend to have migraines, you don't want or need anything stimulating your fifth cranial nerve and your limbic system.

Diagnosing TMD

The first step out of this downward spiral is to begin to connect the dots through my Holistic Dental Matrix. Then find a qualified doctor to be your quarterback and move your health forward.

However, don't let your doctor's lack of knowledge of holistic medicine be a limiting factor to your health. Take an active approach by asking multilevel questions to help your doctor discover the underlying injury or conditions that are causing your problems.

For example, when a tooth becomes painful, you go to the dentist. There, questions are asked and an X-ray is usually taken and the dentist may proclaim, "Everything looks fine. No cavities." Yet if the dentist looks beyond the tooth that is painful to the rest of your mouth, they could see that you have shiny flat areas on your teeth or notches in other teeth near the gum line. Those are clues that something else is going on.

On some people, it's easy to see the effects of tooth grinding. The enamel can get worn down flatly where the teeth are rubbing against each other. Or there might be a small incomplete fracture. Sometimes the cusp of a tooth will break from the pressure of the grinding.

A number of times I've seen the complete vertical fracture of a virgin tooth—without any fillings. Just from the force of biting. That's hardest structure in the human body that was broken against another piece of the hardest structure of the human body!

Other tooth problems that appear are deep notches at the gum line. These semi-circular shaped "lesions" at the base of your teeth aren't caused by bacteria, though sometimes there can be decay in them. Some dentists believe they are caused by abrasion from your toothpaste when you're brushing.[3] I don't; it is more complex than that.

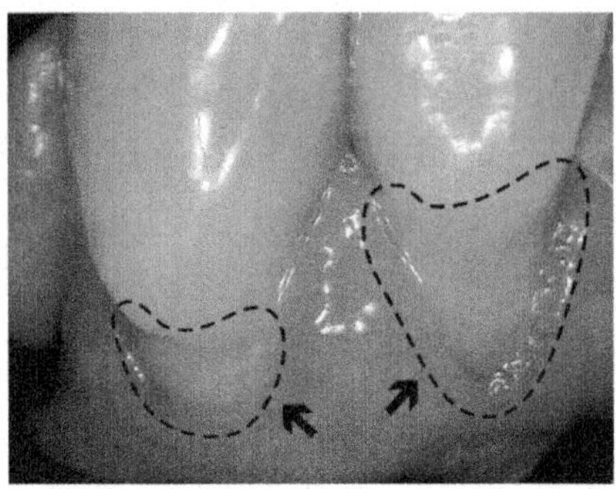

Notches formed by excessive pressure from grinding

I've seen these notches caused by misaligned bite and tooth clenching. Over time, the force of the pressure can cause cracks and splits in the thinnest part of the enamel of your teeth, near the gum line.

These same excessive forces are creating bone loss in your jaw. Grinding damages the tissue of your gums and leads to loose teeth. Then deep pockets can form where bacteria are able to colonize and decay the supporting bone.

When I perform an examination of the muscles in the jaw of someone who grinds their teeth, I can usually feel the tenderness and a pattern begins to emerge. This pain pattern was described by Dr. Janet Travell in her book *Myofascial Pain and Dysfunction: The Trigger Point Manual.*[4] Dr. Travell was President Kennedy's personal physician while he was in the White House. Trigger points are small bunches of contracted muscle fibers. When they are in your jaw, head and neck they can send pain to other areas of your body. They exist in all muscles of your body.

I got the second biggest revelation in my career when I acquired an X-ray device called a Cone Beam Computed Tomography (CBCT for short).This diagnostic device brings together in one fell swoop images of both temporomandibular joints, your nasal passages, sinuses, pharyngeal airway passages and cervical spine as well as various tooth and bone structures.

When I search for the source of migraines, I utilize 3D radiographs of your teeth, jaws, jaw joints and airway. I also look at your medical history, physical exam and biomedical testing. That can include an EMG, transcutaneous electric nerve stimulation (TENS unit), electrosonography (ESG), and computerized mandibular scans (see Diagnosing Sleep Apnea in this chapter).

Safe Treatment

So what can you do once the can of worms has been opened and you've been diagnosed with advanced system/ tissue breakdown in your mouth? The first step of treatment is to decide to take your health into your own hands. *That said, not everyone wants to be "fixed." There are some people who linger in a position of victimhood and don't appreciate it when people try to help them get better*! But I know you are looking for answers or you wouldn't be consulting my Holistic Dental Matrix.

The good news is that your dentist can help treat your TMD and repair your faulty bite by creating an even pressure distribution over all of your biting surfaces. This is accomplished by first and foremost understanding the nature of the problem. Then the following methods can be used: coronoplasty or reshaping the teeth; a removable permanent appliance; permanent restorations on your teeth (i.e. crowns or onlays); orthodontics (if your teeth have enough shape and definition) and lastly surgery, which is a treatment of last resort for most cases of TMD. In fact the incidence in my practice of sending anyone for a surgical consult is less than one person per year.

"Neuromuscular Dentistry" is a term coined by one of my mentors, Dr. Bernard Jankelson, almost 50 years ago. It is the source of some of my greatest joys and successes in treating TMD and bringing those who suffer from it back from the brink. Jankelson developed a philosophy of care and supportive instruments that have withstood the test of time and repeated assaults from those opposed to it. Similar to those found in a religious war.

These principles are applied in both a diagnostic and treatment manner. Part of the treatment is often with a bite balancing device called an orthosis. This is worn on the teeth and may be either fixed to the teeth and not be removed by the patient or removable. Although worn on the teeth, it does not treat the teeth but rather treats the muscles and jaw joint.

The device is carefully constructed for individual use, and is usually worn on your lower teeth. The device is adjusted periodically and evaluated every six weeks or so.

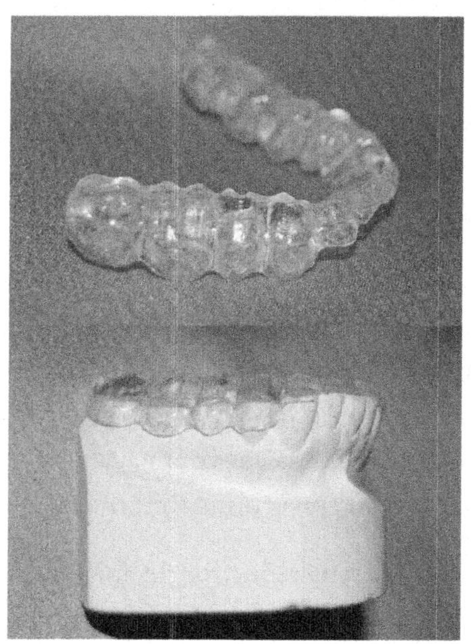

Photos hardly do justice to the refined nature of the orthosis

My treatments are "flavored" or supplemented by additional therapies. These can include trigger point therapy, coupled with Prolozone® treatment. Prolozone involves injections of collagen-producing substances and ozone gas into the damaged connective tissue in and around your muscles and joints.[5] It lessens the pain as it helps the ligaments repair themselves.

Additionally, Craniosacral Therapy (CST) is a gentle, hands-on approach that releases tensions deep in your body to relieve pain and dysfunction and improve whole-body health and performance.[6] It was developed by Osteopathic Physician John E. Upledger after years of clinical testing and research at Michigan State University where he served as professor of biomechanics.

I may also recommend other treatments involving chiropractic adjustments, acupuncture, lymphatic massage, homeopathy, flower essences, or essential oils.

I use some of these same treatments for migraines, but the most successful solution I've found is the FDA-approved Nociceptive Trigeminal Inhibition-Tension Suppression System (NTI-TSS).[7] It's designed to relax the muscles involved in clenching and grinding. The NTI-TSS is a small transparent plastic device that is usually worn over the two front teeth at night (it can also be made for the lower jaw). It keeps your back teeth from coming in contact with each other, preventing the grinding from happening.

I've seen a 70 percent reduction in migraine episodes using the NTI-TSS because it reduces the intensity of the nighttime muscle clenching. A precision orthotic made of clear vinyl can also be worn during the day if your clenching also happens while you're awake.

The great news is that, in my personal experience, you will know if an orthotic device is successful within 30-45 days. In fact, there is most often a vast improvement in your symptoms within the first couple of weeks. Wow—all that with no drugs!

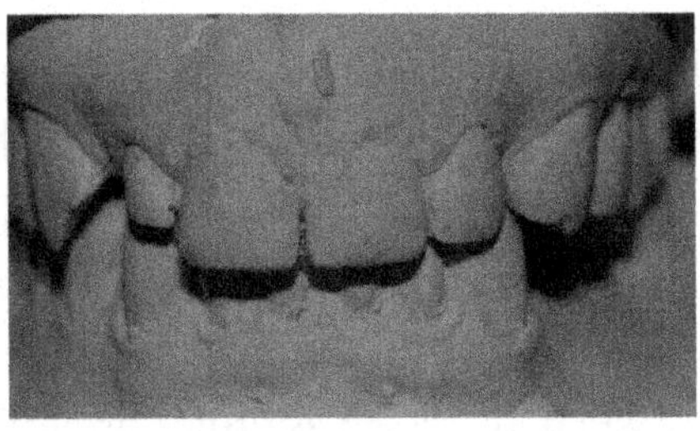

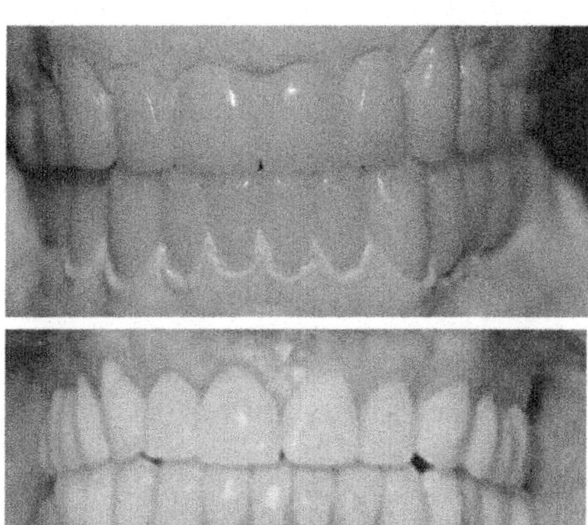

Photo sequence of a successful orthotic adjustment

The following is a letter I received from a patient I helped:

Dear Dr. Meyer,

I am writing to thank and commend you for the quality dental care you have provided for me. Although my dental work has taken a year to complete, the final result has surpassed my expectations and is more than worth the time and expense.

By the time I was in my late 40's I had a mouth of amalgam fillings (mercury), crowns made from a variety of metals as well as several root canals. By my mid 50's my teeth had begun wearing away, breaking and crumbling. After a few more years I began to experience a general decline in health. The toxicity and structural deterioration in my teeth and jaws ultimately proved be a significant contributing cause of the decline in health that I was experiencing.

While I encountered numerous dentists who marketed their practices as "mercury free," it was difficult to find dentists who offered durable and completely metal free solutions to my severe dental issues and it was almost impossible to find dentists with a practical clinical understanding of the complex relationships between the teeth and the other systems and organs of the body. Most dentists I encountered practiced "one tooth at a time" dentistry and seemed to have no sense whatsoever that the different parts of the body significantly influence one another and the body functions as an integral whole.

Unfortunately, my desire to conserve money led me to well recommended dentists in Mexico. While they were able to work at restoring my mouth without metal, as it turned out they too were also practicing "one tooth at a time" dentistry. Within a few years a bridge broke, a crown came off and I started having to go back every year to have overlay restorations repaired or replaced. (You also found active decay under several of their old crowns.) Finally, looking for new solutions to my dental issues, in 2008 I consulted with several new dentists and was told that there was nothing more that could be done to save my teeth. It was recommended that I have all my remaining teeth pulled and get dentures.

I first visited your office in February 2009; I was doubly shocked at the extent of the work you proposed and the anticipated cost. But what you proposed was comprehensive and made good sense. You came up with a plan to save my remaining teeth and you incorporated into your practice an in-depth understanding and appreciation of the critical effect that dental issues can have on general health. We started working together in February 2010.

In February 2011 the work was complete. I now have a full set of teeth that are completely comfortable and fully functional. I can easily eat anything I want. The adjustments that you made to my jaw and bite have allowed me to feel more relaxed and comfortable in my body. You did an excellent job with both implants and crowns and my "new" teeth look far better than my original teeth ever did. You have a gentle and considerate "touch" and I was always comfortable while you were working on me. It always felt like all of the support staff in your office were allies and friends. But, perhaps, best of all you have a depth of experience and expertise that allowed you to plan a course of action that solved the severe dental problems that several other dentists had given up on.

Thank you, Dr. Meyer!

Airway Disorders

Airway disturbances, like so many things, can range from mild to severe. Doctors don't often diagnose the existence of an airway problem just by looking at your teeth and mouth. They have to understand the subtleties and be able to view the structures of your body that are working with and against one another.

To imagine how an airway obstruction works, think of a single car garage (your mouth) and the car (your tongue) that fits in the garage perfectly when you are twelve years old. But as we go through life, we accumulate stuff. We have to put it somewhere so the garage is one of the default places of choice.

When you put a little stuff into the garage, you can still get your car in the garage. But as you accumulate more stuff and store it inside, you can only pull your car in partway so you have to keep the door open.

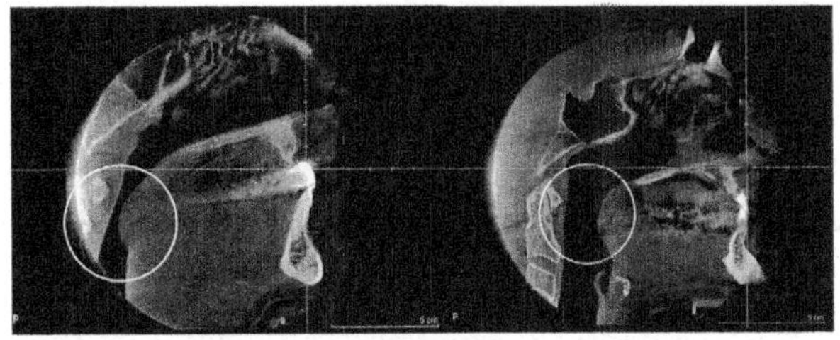

X-ray on left reveals a very "pinched" windpipe, on the right there is exceptional space for air to pass

So what does this garage story have to do with you? We all collect stuff in our bodies like our garage collects our belongings. As we age, our stuff collection can cause inflammation and swelling in the soft tissues of your mouth (see Chapter 2 – Heavy Metal and Chapter 3 – Fluoride). You also lose muscle tone which allows the tissues to collapse. Bone growths can also occur in the mouth. These are akin to pieces of furniture of varying sizes showing up in your garage to crowd out the car (your tongue).

I think you can see where I'm going with this. Just like we don't like keeping our garage door open, we don't like walking around with our tongue hanging out. So we force our tongue back into our mouth to make it look nicer. But now you have a real problem. The car is jammed against your stuff, and you are blocked up. That's what's happening in your mouth, until it gets so bad that you have to do something about it.

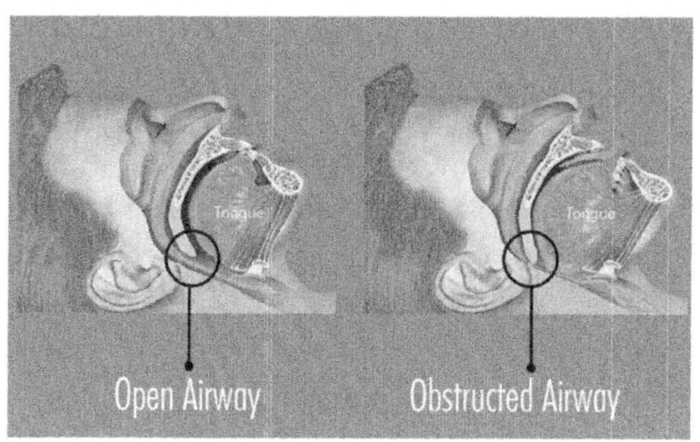

Open airway in the throat vs. an obstructed airway

When your airway is blocked, that interferes with your sleep. According to Greg McKeown, the author of the best seller *Essentialism: The Disciplined Pursuit of Less,* the best asset we have for making a contribution to the world is ourselves. If we under-invest in ourselves, and by that I mean our minds, our bodies and our spirits, then we damage the very tool we need to make our highest contribution. His whole point is getting proper sleep in order to take care of the asset!

You see, Obstructive Sleep Apnea (OSA), snoring, and related sleep disordered breathing conditions lead to varying amounts of the same result—a lack of sleep. The mainstream media is replete with stories of needing adequate sleep for a variety of reasons. Often sleep deprivation involves poor work performance, such as someone falling asleep at the wheel and causing a crash. But the bottom line means taking care of *you*. Sleep, the most essential aspect of our well-being, must not be neglected, overlooked or given the short shrift. It is critical to every aspect of our lives.

TESTIMONY BY R.B.

For many years, my friends and family, fortunate enough to be in proximity of my sleep would tell the wildest tails of a snoring monster. Surely they weren't speaking of me. I never heard this Jekyll/Hyde version of me. It wasn't until I was engaged to my wife did I truly understand how this other being was affecting both my relationship as well as my health.

Reluctantly I took some tests. The findings confirmed the existence of the snoring beast and revealed an issue I never knew about. I was diagnosed with an extremely small windpipe. The testing and development of my appliance was easy. The technology of the solution seemed too simple. Increasing airflow by adjusting my jaw. I was skeptical.

The first few days of using the appliance was odd. Some mild discomfort fueled the notion that if this worked, I would be wearing this forever. But the results were instantaneous. My wife described a night of rest for both of us. The snoring beast had been slain. After about a month, both the discomfort and initial awareness of wearing a mouth piece to bed subsided. And I discovered my ability to fall asleep faster and more soundly increased.

The sleep apnea procedure and appliance has improved my level of quality of rest. It has saved my relationship. It has solved the riddle of the snoring monster. I wish I know known the technology existed earlier.

Sleep Apnea

One of the most serious issues I see with airway problems is sleep apnea. When I'm talking about sleep apnea, I'm referring to Obstructive Sleep Apnea (OSA), the most common kind of apnea that people suffer from. The other type is Central Sleep Apnea, which occurs because your brain doesn't send proper signals to the muscles that control your breathing. That is a more serious condition and fortunately it's much less common than OSA. These conditions are diagnosed by a physician who has special interest in sleep disorders. It can be a sleep medicine specialist, pulmonologist, neurologist, PhD psychologist or other physicians.

With obstructive sleep apnea, your brain sends a signal to breathe but because of an obstruction of your airway, your breathing stops for 10 seconds, 20 seconds or even more. These breathless episodes (apneas) may occur many times during the night. In essence, you are suffocating intermittently throughout the night.

Sleep apnea is commonly accompanied by snoring but not always. Snoring is caused by a narrowing of your upper airway, which leads to the vibration of your throat (pharyngeal) tissues. This is considered to be a partial obstruction of the airway, whereas with sleep apnea there is a full obstruction of the airway.

Go to my website for a short video on snoring and sleep apnea, or access it directly here:

Sleep apnea is a very serious problem. If you have sleep apnea, you have an increased risk of: heart disease, stroke, diabetes, depression, anxiety, high blood pressure, pulmonary hypertension, congestive heart failure and coronary artery disease. I also see massive destruction in teeth with deposits of bone that are probably linked to sleep apnea.

When you have sleep apnea, two things are going wrong in your body. You aren't getting enough sleep because you keep having to wake up to breathe (sleep deprivation). Plus you're not getting enough oxygen (hypoxia) for your system because you stop breathing. The common medical answer to these issues is the Continuous Positive Airway Pressure device more commonly called a CPAP.

There is a fairly broad range or span between what is considered healthy/normal and OSA. Certainly, the closer you are to the actual threshold number needed to be said that you have OSA, the greater the damage that can be done. So what about the person who has been seen by a sleep physician on the suspicion of OSA, and their numbers aren't quite within the range of diagnosing OSA? The final word is, *no* OSA! Even if they have numbers that are just shy of the trigger number to be officially classified.

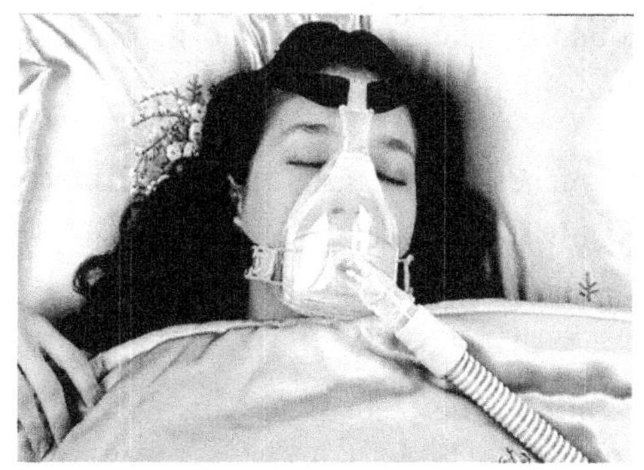

Sleep apnea sufferer wearing a CPAP device

However dental woes surface long before the actual by-the-numbers diagnosis of OSA, such as fractured teeth, periodontal disease caused by the physical overload, pH imbalance and other issues. Our medical and dental systems let these folk languish in a veritable no man's land without a definitive recognition of their ongoing problem. With no official name as to what you have, you are pronounced "normal" so you have to go about your business until the next tooth breaks or your spouse might catch you gasping for breath at night, or you suffer a stroke or heart attack from low oxygen.

The physiology of lack of sleep and lack of oxygen is so entwined they can only be artificially separated for the sake of discussion. But really they aren't separable. We sleep for a lot of different reasons, including health repair and restoration during that down time. We also need to have oxygen coming into our body at all times. This is especially a problem at night because our muscle tone is much lower. That means the soft tissue of your throat can collapse. The healthier one is, the greater the tone remains through the night.

One of the biggest problems is that lack of oxygen alters the pH (potential Hydrogen) of your body. This is supposed to be 7.35-7.45 for humans. When our body perceives the slightest lowering from this level, feedback signals let your body know of the need to "buffer" the change and bring your blood back to 7.35-7.45. The minerals needed for this come from our bones and it happens in microseconds. It is a real time system that keeps constant watch for any change that takes place.

So when your pH is constantly shifting from lack of oxygen, it stresses your entire body. We've already talked about the effect your fight or flight response has on your body when you are constantly stressed. Like TMD, sleep apnea is a condition that takes its toll on you a little more every day. Two major studies have found that sleep apnea causes so much damage to your body that it can shorten your life by years.[8]

The Physics of Breathing

It's important for you to know that there is solid science behind these air flow dynamics. The following is presented for those of you who like mathematical equations. For those that want to skip this part, jump down to the second to last paragraph of this section.

The equation for laminar flow is expressed in Poiseulle's law, in which the pressure (P) difference between the two ends of a tube through which there is a flow is directly proportional to the volume flowing per unit time (Q), to the viscosity of the fluid (v), to the length of the tube (L) and inversely related to the fourth power of the radius:

$$P_1 - P_2 = Q8LV/2\pi r^2$$

It is apparent from this equation that pressure is extremely sensitive to radius. A 2-fold decrease in radius of an airway, for example, requires a 16-fold increase in pressure if the flow is to remain constant.

The relationship between pressure and flow in the presence of turbulence is exponential, pressure being related not simply to the velocity of flow but to the square of velocity, e.g., doubling the flow requires a fourfold increase in pressure:

$$P_1 - P_2 = KQ^2$$

So in real simple terms, if you suffer the loss of half the circumference of your windpipe, you will require a 16 fold increase of pressure to deliver the same amount of oxygen.

The narrower the tube (more obstructed), the greater the resistance. So little changes yield big results, both good and bad. And I promise you there will be no more equations.

Diagnosing Sleep Apnea

Dentists are often considered to be the best physicians to treat snoring and sleep apnea because of our familiarity with the prosthetic devices used in treatment. Diagnosis and treatment often go hand in hand with sleep apnea.

Go to my website for a simple screening test for Obstructive Sleep Apnea: www.DrNicholasMeyer.com.

After a bona fide sleep study that confirms the presence of OSA, the tool I use next is Acoustic Reflection Rhinometry.[9] It's a noninvasive technique that sends a sound pulse through your nose. The sound waves bounce off the tissues inside your nose and return to the sending source where a sensor picks up the signals. The information is displayed on a computer monitor, giving me a clear view of obstructions in your nasal passages.

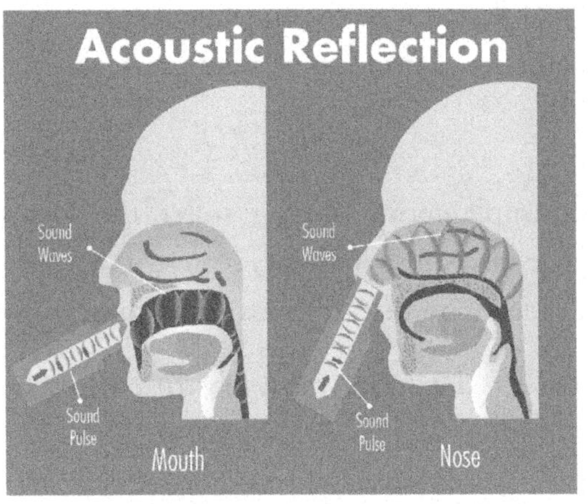

Diagnosing the size of the airway

I also use Acoustic Reflection Pharyngometry, which sends the same sort of sound pulse and reflection to map out the interior of your mouth.[10] This kind of sound wave doesn't hurt your tissues, and it's very easy to do in my office.

Once I can see what your interior structures look like, I know where the location of the problem is. The bonus is that I can use the images to pick a jaw position that will create the most open airway for you.

Another tool I use for diagnosing soft tissue disorders is 3D X-ray scanning. This innovation has advanced the field of dental medicine over the past decade by showing us the structures of your teeth and jaw in 3D instead of flat images.

A number of different companies make 3D X-ray scanners, from smaller units to more complex ones. Some minimal units show only a small segment of your teeth. These devices are typically used in the field of endodontics (root canal therapy).

The next level of scanner includes the imaging of your jaws but only one side or the other. These are typically used by doctors who are placing dental implants, but they aren't necessarily useful for diagnosing TMD or airway obstructions.

But the highest level of 3D scanning has fantastic capabilities and a much larger functionality. I can use my 3D scanner to image your jaw joints, upper neck, sinuses, nasal and pharyngeal airways—the whole enchilada. I have successfully used my unit for almost a decade, and the information that it provides is invaluable.

With the click of the button or the spin of the scroll wheel on my computer mouse, I can see in action how everything in your mouth, jaw and throat are working together simultaneously. This tool removed any doubt I had that all of your structures are interrelated in a dynamic balance, and the consequences of imbalances in your system can be seen if you look in the right place.

To see a video of 3D scanning, go to my website www.DrNicholasMeyer.com or use this QR code:

Safe Treatment

Treatment obviously depends on what the cause of the malady is. One question to answer is: Can this problem be solved completely or can this problem only be managed?

One way that I treat sleep apnea involves the use of dental appliances. Oral Appliance Therapy (OAT) works on a simple premise: if you can control the position of your jaw or the posture of your tongue, then you can control (for the most part) the volume of air that enters your airway.

There are now over 100 OAT devices on the market with more being developed. The goal for all of them is the same: to help you breathe at night. It's almost like a journey by car, where you have the option to take a Volkswagen, a Buick or a Ferrari to your destination. The question is, how efficiently do you want to get there?

Most doctors will learn a few appliances really well, so they can deliver good service that is predictable and comfortable. I see a custom appliance as highly individualized care, tailored to the specific needs of your body. I also know that some people may need supplemental help in the form of dental implants that provide anchorage to keep the device in place.

Are these devices for everyone? No! Some people's problems aren't suited for oral appliance therapy. If a patient isn't sure it will work for them, I will sometimes suggest that they buy an over-the-counter device first prior to getting a custom one made. It's not ideal, but not everyone is interested in "ideal." They just want some relief and to be able to sleep at night. Still others are best suited for the traditional CPAP device.

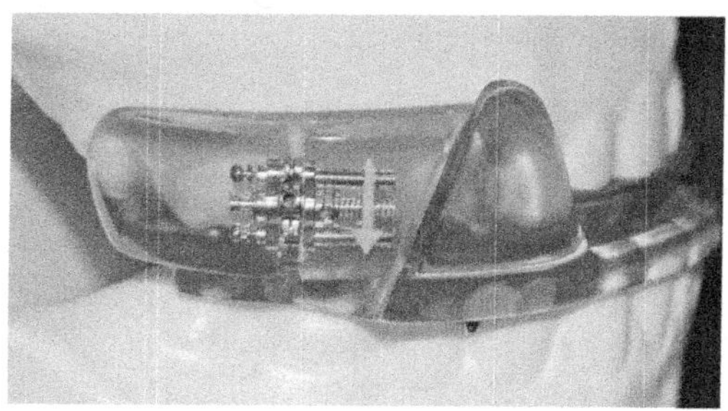

This appliance is for both upper jaw and lower jaw and is comfortable to wear

I believe in allowing people to rise to the level of health that they aspire to. If, after a successful or an unsuccessful trial with a store bought device, they are ready to try a custom device, then the next step is measuring using the diagnostic instruments previously described. This allows me to figure out anatomical considerations that guide the decision as to which device is better suited to manage the conditions that are present.

Sometimes oral appliance therapy needs to give way to the removal of the oral obstacles in your airway. You can see in the photo on the following page that this patient has extraordinarily large bone growths (non-cancerous) in the floor of their mouth that altered tongue posture and function.

These growths needed to be cleared out to make room for the airway. As an aside, these severely sized growths occur most often in those individuals that have extremely hard teeth. It is as if the forces from grinding are not absorbed by the tooth but transmitted right through the tooth. This stimulates the periosteum (first layer of tissue that covers any bone) to create more bone.

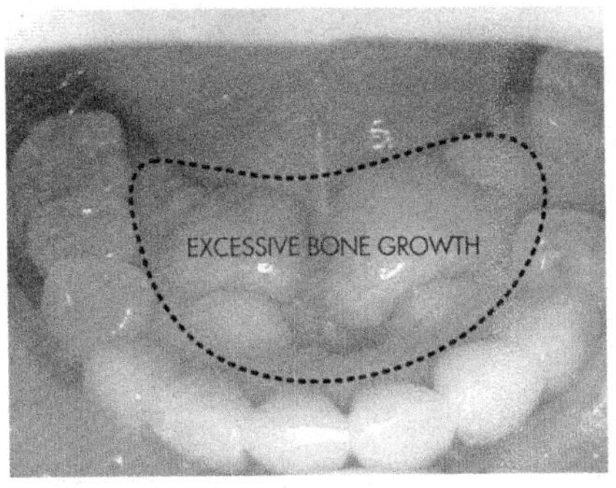

Bone growths obstruct the airway by crowding the tongue

The primary mainstream treatments that are used to help people with obstructive sleep apnea include the CPAP (and all of its iterations) and several surgical techniques. For example, there is one surgery, the Tonsillar Pillar that stiffens a floppy uvula.[11] Small, stiff fiberglass-like rods are inserted into the uvula to prop it up, making it less flaccid so you can maintain a more open airway.

The uvulopalatopharyngoplasty (UUUP or UP3) is an even more invasive surgery.[12] Here the soft tissue drape of the throat, that includes the uvula, is removed so that there is nothing left to vibrate and thus cause noise. I am sure that there are people who have been helped by this procedure, but in my personal experience, I haven't seen any of them. In fact the breathing issue is usually unaffected as the underlying problem in the collapse of the soft tissue has not been identified and corrected by the surgery.

CASE STUDY

JS was one of my patients who suffered from sleep apnea. He was in his mid-60s and he had already had many medical treatments before I saw him that didn't help him. One of worst was the throat surgery that removed his uvula. He came to see me for dental care because his current dental apparatuses weren't working.

When I examined him, I saw there was a deficiency of support in his lower jaw that caused him to look prematurely old. When I properly aligned his jaws, his airway opened up. He was then able to sleep much better through the night and he regained a more youthful appearance in his face. He went from 2-3 hours of sleep per night to 6-7 hours.

He writes, "This was a major project and I had the finest Dr. and staff... My new dental work turned out just like Dr. Meyer designed it and it is beautiful. It was a joy to come in for treatments."

Life style modification is one of the absolute best ways to help yourself, including a fat management program. It is the white belly fat that harms us. It is difficult to achieve health, but it's oh so necessary. In addition to helping to self-treat sleep apnea, you can see other changes occurring. For instance, there is a high likelihood that your lipid (fat) profile will improve, your blood sugar will normalize and you will significantly take yourself out of the danger zone of crossing over in the Type II Diabetes world and all of those troubles.

Airway Issues in Childhood

Children with airway problems are at a high risk of becoming adults with sleep apnea disease. This is an area of keen interest in the dental community because there is a much greater awareness of the lifelong disability that these youngsters face. Without care, these children who are afflicted will grow up into an adult with problems. These problems aren't just an airway disturbance but will be system wide.

The adaptations that these little people have to make will be with them their whole life and of course will be exacerbated when they get older. In my own case, I had tonsil problems (think airway), that required I have them removed at age 5. Shortly afterwards I developed exercise induced asthma. I had a recessed or retruded jaw and as I grew up my need for air caused me to compensate posturally and I developed a forward head posture. I was a mess. Today, I have a slight forward head posture (I have worked hard to correct it) and a repostured lower jaw, thanks to a forward thinking orthodontist when in high school.

A variety of orthopedic (bone changing) removable and fixed appliances are also used to treat children who have imbalances of the head, neck and upper airway. The field today is known as Airway Orthodontics (see Chapter 12 – Holistic Dental Resources). The most common problem is that of undeveloped jaws, both upper jaw and lower jaw. These are easily seen and recognized in children if the primary focus isn't on the cosmetic issues of the teeth position alone.

The child's dentist needs to be aware of the problems that are caused by a diminished airway, demonstrated, in part, by small jaws. In children from age 2-11 years old, a good sign to see is spaces between the upper teeth from side to side and the lower front teeth from side to side.

The traditional answer for crowded teeth for many dentists is to remove teeth. Because the jaw is too small for them all to fit. But the answer isn't in removing the teeth to make the small jaw accommodate the teeth, but rather to grow the jaw three-dimensionally to accommodate the teeth.

The use of orthopedic appliances can "develop" the size and the shape of their jaws to a much more desirable state. This might take a longer time than simply pulling teeth, but it is far better to get the jaw size on track while the bones are so malleable and then wait for the teeth to come in. Later, fixed appliances like braces can help with minor tweaking. It's not the perfect solution, but it is far better than condemning the child to a lifetime of airway troubles as an adult.

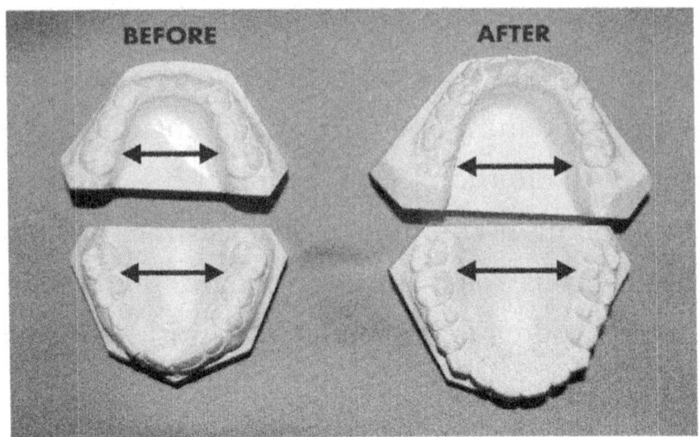

These models are of the same child: The "Arch Development" treatment successfully enlarged the child's jaw on the right.

Conclusion

The Holistic Dental Matrix approach contributes to your overall health in a way that traditional medicine does not when it comes to TMD and airway disorders. That's why holistic dentistry can enhance your health and well-being while fixing the real problem in your teeth, jaw and mouth. If you don't pay attention to these basic principles, all kinds of illness can manifest, sometimes years down the line, seriously compromising your health.

End Notes

[1] "TMJ Disorders." *TMJ Disorders*. National Institute of Dental and Craniofacial Research. Web. 25 Feb. 2016.

[2] "Jaw Tension - The Migraine Trust." *The Migraine Trust*. Web. 26 Feb. 2016.

[3] Sadaf, D. and Z. Ahmad. "Role of Brushing and Occlusal Forces in Non-Carious Cervical Lesions (NCCL)." *Int J Biomed Sci.* 10.4 (December 2014): 265–268.

[4] Wilson, V.P. "Janet G. Travell, MD: A Daughter's Recollection." *Tex Heart Inst J*. 30.1 (2003): 8–12.

[5] Elvis, A.M. and J.S. Ekta. "Ozone therapy: A clinical review." *J Nat Sci Biol Med.* 2.1 (Jan-June 2011): 66–70.

[6] "Discover CranioSacral Therapy." *Discover CranioSacral Therapy*. Web. 26 Feb. 2016.

[7] Stapelmann, H. and J.C. Türp. "The NTI-tss device for the therapy of bruxism, temporomandibular disorders, and headache – Where do we stand? A qualitative systematic review of the literature." *BMC Oral Health* 8.22 (2008).

[8] "Sleep Apnea Wakes up Heart Disease - Harvard Health." *The Family Health Guide*. Harvard Health Publications, 2008. Web. 26 Feb. 2016.

[9] Clement, P.A.R. and F. Gordts. "Consensus report on acoustic rhinometry and rhinomanometry." *Rhinology* 43.3 (2005): 169-.

[10] Gelardi, M., A.M. del Giudice, F. Cariti, M. Cassano, A.C. Farras, M.L. Fiorella and P. Cassano. "Acoustic pharyngometry: clinical and instrumental correlations in sleep disorders." *Rev Bras Otorrinolaringol* 73.2 (2007): 257-65.

[11] Chan, J., L.M. Akst, and I. Eliachar. "The roles of the anterior tonsillar pillar and previous tonsillectomy on sleep-disordered breathing." *Ear Nose Throat J.* 83.6 (June 2004): 408-413.

[12] Khan, A., K. Ramar, S. Maddirala, O. Friedman, J.F. Pallanch and E.J. Olson. "Uvulopalatopharyngoplasty in the Management of Obstructive Sleep Apnea: The Mayo Clinic Experience." *Mayo Clin Proc.* 84.9 (Sept 2009): 795–800.

CHAPTER 5

ROOT CANALS & JAW BONE LESIONS: HIDDEN CAUSES OF DISEASE

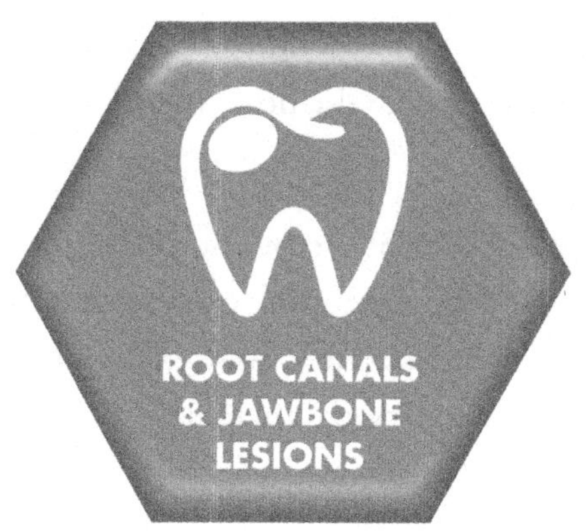

When you look at my Holistic Dental Matrix™, some of the symptoms that can bring you to this chapter may look very different from each other. But believe me, there is a common source for all of these health problems.

You could be having headaches: either cluster type headaches or pain under your eyes from your maxillary sinus. Or you could have trigeminal neuralgia, a chronic pain condition that affects the trigeminal or 5th cranial nerve, which stimulates your flight or fight response. With excessive nerve stimulation, you can also get cold sores (herpes simplex type 1) as a symptom.

You might also be experiencing pain in your face that is atypical, which means the pain is vague and you're not sure what is causing it.

Or you may be having heart symptoms such as an abnormal tachycardia, when your heart beats too fast at more than 100 beats per minute. You may have had an abnormal Electrocardiograph (EKG), abnormally high blood pressure or cardiomyopathy, which is a condition where the heart muscle is abnormal.

You also might have something known as mitochondrial dysfunction, which is a failure of your cells to produce enough energy to sustain life.[1] That can cause a number of systemic diseases. This is on the rise due to multiple causes but one notable cause is that of environmental factors. It is believed that it is a secondary effect to these factors.

Also, with jaw bone cavitations (tissue damage or lesions in the bone of your jaw) you may get seemingly unrelated symptoms such as kidney pain, bladder pain, back pain, chronic fatigue and chemical sensitivity.

In this chapter, I've put root canals and jaw bone lesions/ cavitations together because the source of your health problems throughout your body may be found in the altered tissue of your mouth. This damaged tissue reacts by releasing toxic chemicals into your body. This is what is known as the toxicology of these disease entities. In my experience, jaw bone cavitations are approximately five times more toxic than root canals.

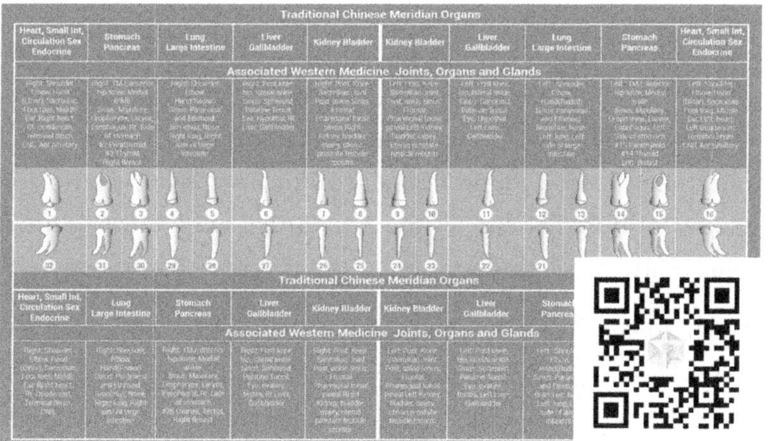

This dental meridian chart shows which organs are energetically affected by toxins in your teeth or jaw bone. Clearly toxins know no boundaries when it comes to making your body ill. This chart is an adaptation by Drs. Louisa Williams and Dietrich Klinghardt. The full chart may be seen at end of Chapter 1, or use QR code above to see interactive version.

Root Canals

Root canal! A term that is known to strike fear into the hearts of men and women. It is a procedure that is performed with the intention to "save a tooth." One that has been painful or rotted or somehow no longer healthy. Root canal treatment basically consists of a doctor removing the fine little nerve bundle (either alive or not) from inside of the tooth. This renders the tooth "non-vital". We say they are not dead but without the blood supply to the tooth one can only wonder what it is then.

If you've had one or more root canals done in the past it may be causing or contributing to some systemic health problems today, including fibromyalgia, chronic inflammation and bacterial infections. Teeth with root canals treatments contain dozens and dozens of different species of bacteria that are known to affect your heart, nerves, kidneys, brain, sinus cavities and more.

The toxicity of root canals was discovered by doctors at the Mayo Clinic and Dr. Weston Price a hundred or so years ago. Dr. Price's book published in 1922 revealed extensive documentation of the transmissibility of disease from a human to a rabbit when a tooth with a root canal was placed under the skin of a rabbit. While Dr. Price was the head of research for the now-defunct National Dental Association (predecessor to the current American Dental Association), he attempted to sterilize 1,000 extracted teeth, but 990 of the teeth cultured toxic bacteria just two days after treatment with chemicals designed to make the tooth sterile.[2]

Even conventional dentistry agrees that root canal teeth have an inflammatory marker known as Tumor Necrosis Factor alpha (TNFa) in the bone tissue adjacent to the teeth.[3] This and other inflammatory markers have no business being next to "healthy" teeth. They can only be found there if the area is under biochemical stress.

Furthermore, when we are trying to figure out why these types of markers are present, we have to think beyond our traditional ideas of infection as a bacterial overload and begin to think more in terms of a toxic overload on your body.

What happens is that a root canal can trap bacteria within the small microtubules in your teeth. Connected to the main channel within the center of the tooth, there are microtubules that jut out sideways into the area of the ligament where your tooth attaches to the bone. Trapped bacteria in your teeth may spread into the surrounding boney tissue.

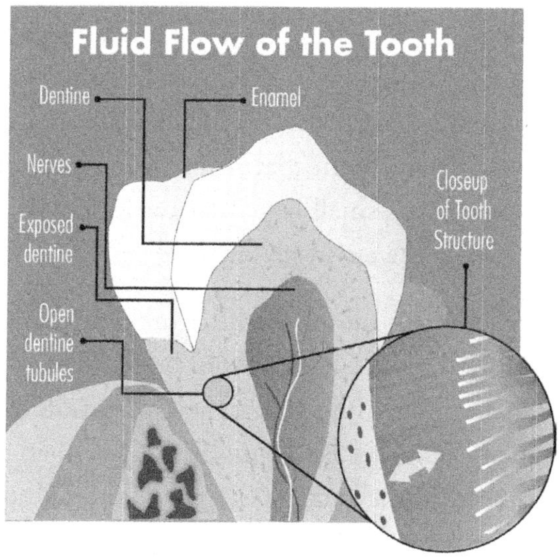

Microtubules can carry bacteria
into the surrounding bone

When a tooth is healthy, the circulatory system within it causes a positive pressure gradient. That means that fluid flows from within the closed chamber of your tooth under relatively high pressure to move slowly out through the small tubules and into the surrounding ligaments in the space around your tooth.

Researchers Drs. Leonora and Steinman, of Loma Linda University, identified this positive pressure gradient or "perspiration" that keeps the tooth clean by flushing acids and bacteria from the enamel.[4] It was found to be under the control of Parotid Hormone. But when sugar is eaten, this pump mechanism goes into reverse and instead of flushing the acids and bacteria out and away; the tooth actually sucks the acids and bacteria into the microtubules.

When a tooth dies for whatever reason, including when a root canal is done on it to remove the living pulp, that positive fluid pressure stops and we have what is known as stasis or stagnation. This is akin to a beaver dam that stops up a stream, causing a backup of water into a small bay. That causes stagnation and a complete change in the environment.

For your tooth, this means the little tubules turn into a nice hiding place for bacteria that are in your body. When the bacteria take up residence inside these tubes, they are outside the reach of your immune system and the white blood cells that are present to fight infection. So the bacteria can grow and multiply there.

As the bacteria grow, the oxygen is used up in the area so it changes from an oxygen-rich environment to an oxygen-poor environment. So then the bacteria have to change their metabolism. They go from what is called aerobic (oxygen-using) to anaerobic (oxygen shunning). When bacteria are in the anaerobic phase, they create substances known as endotoxins.

These endotoxins are what damage your body. Toxins are proteins and are free to move around your body. So the toxins are pumped out of the diseased tissue by your circulatory system and travel throughout your body.

CASE STUDY

A woman in her late 50s came to me complaining about a medical condition known as interstitial cystitis. This is a painful inflammatory condition of the bladder. People who have this feel an urgency to void the bladder all of the time because urine irritates the lining.

After consulting with me, the woman decided to have all of her root canal teeth removed—four altogether. Within six weeks, her bladder inflammation was gone and she was able to go back to a normal lifestyle. We then restored her mouth with removable partial dentures. The 4 teeth that were removed were not on what is known as the kidney/bladder meridian (top and bottom front four teeth). However toxins from root canal teeth know no specific boundaries or limitations.

Diagnosing Root Canal Problems

First, the way to discover whether root canals might be causing your problems is to be open to the idea that they can. It's sometimes hard to realize that what's happening in your body may be caused by your root canal.

It's not always easy to diagnose root canal problems using routine diagnostic tools such as X-ray analysis, but tools such as Autonomic Response Testing (ART) and electro acupuncture or EAV/EDS can work. Often having some other health care coach can be helpful here.

Autonomic response testing and "muscle testing" is based on the phenomenon that a muscle will become weak when some type of interference is encountered. I test both points—your tooth and the problem area—to see if they are linked. If you are interested, you can find a great deal more information and in-depth discussion of this type of bio-feedback phenomenon online.

A relatively recent test using DNA probe analysis called PCR (polymerase chain reaction) can identify dozens of different bacterial species that can be harvested from your tooth (or any tissue that you might be concerned about). This is accomplished rather easily by taking a sterile paper point that is about a half inch long. It is placed into the small crevice that is between the tooth and the outer surface of the gum tissue of the tooth that needs to be sampled. There is a fluid, like lymph, that comes up from around the neck of the tooth. This fluid is captured and then sent for analysis. The lab sends back a report in a few days that indicates what the bacterial forms are and how they can be related to some of the health challenges that you either do have or could have as a result of having these bugs in your mouth.

These teeth, by the way, can be asymptomatic (meaning without symptoms) but the patient suffers ill health. The test results reveal the multitude of bacteria and other lifeforms that are associated with teeth that are by considered by some standards as "clinically healthy." For more information about the nature of these organisms, please see: www.DrNicholasMeyer.com.

So where do these bacterial forms come from? Well, it isn't the tooth fairy! I do subscribe to the scientific premise of pleomorphism. We know that bacterial precursors and other bacteria are floating around our body at all times. When they find a hospitable environment for their optimal well-being, they take up residence. They flourish based on the local environment. However, as the environment changes they do as well. This is also true of a biofilm.

The fact that your body is more interlinked than science originally thought is now well-known by researchers. At the inaugural meeting of the Society of Oxidative and Photonic Medicine in Utah in June, 2015, triple board-certified medical doctor Zachary Bush emphatically stated that root canals are associated with cancer. He performed an analysis of his own patient population, and identified that a root canal on an upper first molar was present in 85 percent of his patients who had breast cancer.[5]

Several years ago, Dr. Thomas Rau told a similar story of his findings. Dr. Rau operates the Paracelsus clinics in Switzerland. He asserted that the number of breast cancer patients with a root canal on an upper first molar was close to 100 percent in his analysis.[6]

More recently, Dr. Jerry Tennant released his new book on cancer: *Healing is Voltage: Cancer's On/Off Switches: Polarity.* Dr. Tennant emphatically asserts that diseased teeth are related to 90 percent or more of cancers.

The reason is because the tooth treated by root canal "shorts out" the electrical circuitry of the body that pertains to the meridian as outlined by Chinese medicine. A meridian is the part of our body that is like circuitry, carrying the energy and signals from one part of your body to another. These are actual structures within the body that follow what are called the fascial planes. Thus a meridian or electric wire that is adversely affected by a tooth will then have some type of trouble within the system.

Safe Treatment

A holistic dentist will look at other options when a patient's problem traditionally calls for a root canal. You have to take into account which tooth is involved, and you also have to take into account your medical doctor's opinion. It can really become a complex issue depending on your situation.

How we solve these problems with root canal teeth really depends on your symptoms. If you have pain without any other health issues, I can inject ozone gas directly into the tissue and that is highly effective for eliminating pain.

If you are having other health issues, often the best solution is to remove the root canal tooth, and create partial dentures or "flipper" to replace the tooth or teeth.

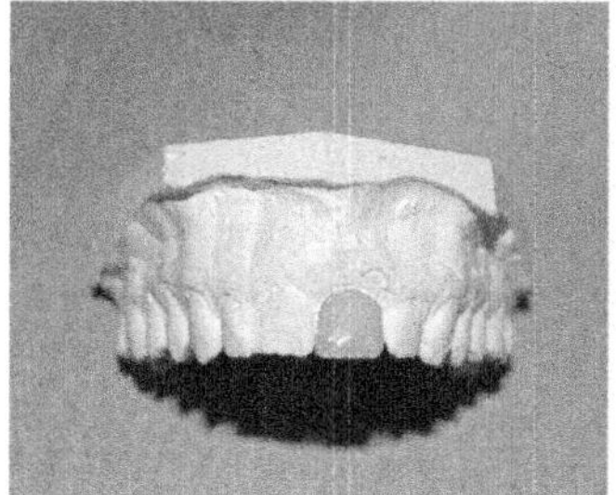
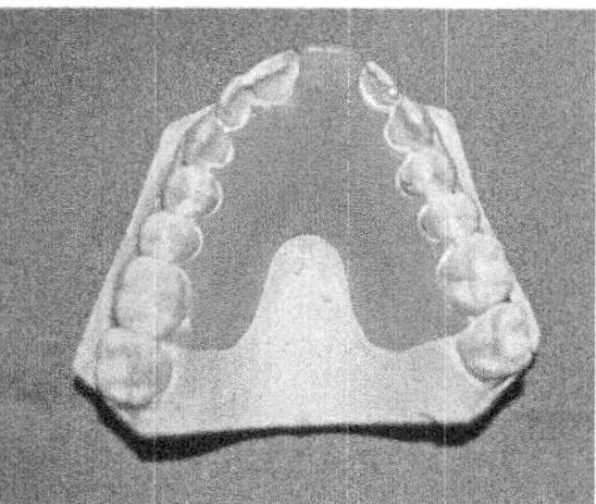

An example of a flipper

We also have a new treatment at our disposal to use on root canals that treats the tissues of your gum and the root of your tooth. The technique known as photon induced photoacoustic streaming (PIPS for short) was developed by a dentist in Scottsdale, Arizona. This version of laser assisted root canal therapy uses a beam of low energy, intense light to clean away the diseased tissues, bacteria and infection better than traditional treatments. Since the clean-out is so effective, healing takes less time and there is less post-operative pain. This can be a viable option to retain a troubled tooth when the other options are less viable.

CASE STUDY

A female patient in her early 60s had a root canal tooth on her upper left lateral incisor, the tooth that is one off-center to the left from your upper front teeth. The problem she was having seemed completely unrelated—her internal organs hurt on that side of her body. After a lengthy consultation with me, she decided to have the tooth removed. Within a matter of weeks all of her pain disappeared. She was wearing a small removable dental prosthetic device known as a "flipper."

Several months later she went to a specialist who inserted a titanium dental implant to replace the incisor so that she wouldn't have to wear her flipper. Within weeks after the implant was placed, the same symptoms that she had previously returned. At first she didn't connect the dots. She returned to the specialist who had placed her implant, only to hear, "There is nothing wrong that I can see." Upon consultation with me once again, she decided to remove the dental implant. After the implant was removed, her symptoms completely disappeared once again. So now today, years later, she still wears her flipper. She remains symptom free.

For children who have had extensive cavities yet they need to maintain the spacing involving the damaged tooth, I suggest a partial root canal treatment instead of a root canal. This can allow the blood flow to be intact into the tooth. Fortunately, the child will be losing this tooth in the not so distant future. This treatment is best accomplished through the use of laser root canal therapy. Thus the tooth can be retained in function and to hold the place for the developing permanent tooth. Other agents have been used in traditional dentistry but they are toxic to your nervous system. Their names are Formocresol or some derivation. This substance has been shown to travel from the tooth to the brain.

Jaw Bone Lesions or Cavitations

A cavity is a hole, so in a tooth we call the hard tissue infection a cavity and this is what you get drilled out and filled. A cavitation is the common term within dentistry for a hole in your bone. A jaw bone cavitation is a hole that contains dead or dying bone and bacterial infection, both of which release toxins into your body. The hole is hard to detect because it can't be seen in the mouth with the unaided eye and it doesn't show up well on x-rays, nor does it cause redness, swelling or fever.[7]

The term "cavitation" was first used to describe a lesion that forms when the blood supplying oxygen is shut off due to the spread of toxins. This results in the death of the bone tissue and a hole or hollowed out portion of the jaw. Dr. G.V. Black (the Father of Modern Dentistry and Dean of the dental school at Northwestern University in Chicago) saw and wrote about this condition as early as 1915, and five years later he named it Neuralgia Inducing Cavitational Osteonecrosis (NICO).[8]

The term NICO is used today when you have symptoms of severe facial pain, neuralgia, headache or a phantom toothache. Although jaw bone cavitations are a common problem, fortunately only a small percentage of people suffer from pain. However, when people do have pain, because cavitations aren't well known, they often seek help from a number of doctors in the hopes of finding a solution.

Jaw bone cavitations may be caused by a form of bacteria that is antibiotic resistant and adheres to your blood vessels. Toxins and by-products from the bacteria create the damaged tissue.

Research has shown that these toxins can combine with chemicals or heavy metals, such as mercury, forming even more potent toxins. German toxicologists have found that the jaw bone can be a biological reservoir for chemicals and heavy metals.[9]

The following is a cut-away view of the inside of a lower jaw bone. The blackish color is the decayed bone.

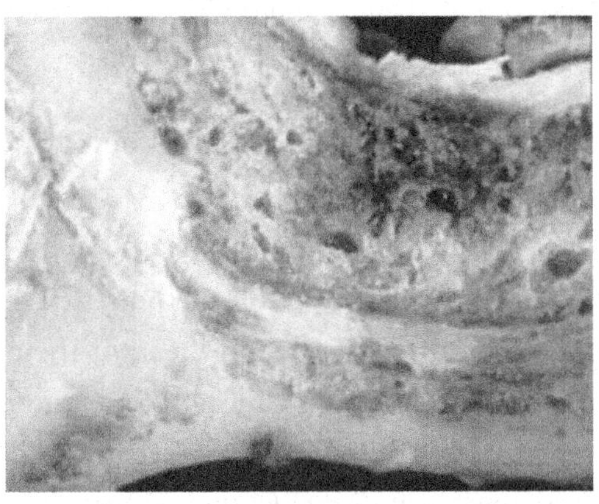

Photograph of a jaw bone cavitation

Cavitations are often found in places where your teeth have been pulled, particularly your wisdom teeth. It's estimated that 45 percent of all jaw bone cavitations are located in your third molar area where your wisdom teeth have been extracted.[10] These areas are more vulnerable because they contain the small terminal (end) blood vessels (called the microvasculature) and bone death (cavitation) is the consequence of injury to these microscopic vessels. The injury can be lack of oxygen (anoxia) or toxins from bacteria or protein breakdown products. This is very similar to the medical condition called CCSVI or Chronic Cerebrospinal Venous Insufficiency. This condition is when there is normal flow into the cerebrospinal fluid but there is a very poor outflow resulting in stagnation and back up. This is a marvelous recipe for illness caused by bacterial infection.

Cavitations are also found under or near the roots of teeth that have had a root canal, or under teeth that are considered to be dead (avital).

We know that cavitations progressively impair the blood supply to the bone marrow in your jaw, which can result in more bone death (osteonecrosis). The damaged tissue may spread throughout your jaw bone, penetrating your sinuses, and even surrounding your inferior jaw nerve (alveolar).

When you take a tissue sample from a cavitation, it always contains toxins that significantly inhibit one or more of the enzymes used in the energy production cycle (the Krebs cycle).

When the Krebs cycle is impeded at any point, it is said to be impaired (mitochondrial dysfunction). The production of energy in your cells can come to a halt or "dysregulated." That energy is what powers you in your day-to-day life. If you have poor energy production, then you will have chronic fatigue. Cavitations have been associated with chronic fatigue by researchers.[11]

To make matters worse, this process affects the local blood supply in your jaw bone, which makes the cavitation spread even further.

Some cavitations aren't caused by extracted teeth or a root canal. Sometimes a tooth never develops, and the bud is the seed that can set off the decaying in your jaw. Most people get their wisdom teeth around age 18. But I regularly hear patients say, "I was lucky, I only got two of my four wisdom teeth." In my mind, I wonder how lucky were they? What happened in their body that caused the death of the tooth bud? What happened to the corpse of that bud?

I have seen numerous times that the site of a wisdom tooth that did not develop is the problem. That unresolved tissue is a source of chronic irritation and toxicity, so I have to surgically remove the tissue that once upon a time was destined to become a wisdom tooth.

A colleague from Munich, Germany, Dr. Johann Lechner, has been researching the relationship of these degenerative osteopathies (bone diseases) and silent inflammation in the jaw bone. His results are quite convincing that there is an intimate relationship of the common dental treatments, i.e. root canal fillings and the removal of wisdom teeth, to the development of inflammatory mediators (little messengers between the cells) and the risk of acquiring some type of immunological and systemic/neurodegenerative disease like cancer or autoimmune diseases, inflammation, arthritis and disorders of the central nervous system (CNS).

Diagnosing Cavitations

In order to diagnose these types of bony lesions, the doctor must understand the subtle nature of this kind of damaged bone tissue. Additionally your doctor needs to know the different types of symptoms, some seemingly unrelated to your teeth that would lead them to examine you for these types of lesions. By cross-referencing the Holistic Dental Matrix you can see how many symptoms are connected with cavitations.

When I suspect there is a jaw bone cavitation, I often use Autonomic Response Testing (ART) to help diagnose them in the same way I use it to diagnose problems associated with root canals. It's a useful and relatively easy-to-administer test.

Another way that I diagnose jaw bone cavitations is through the use of a panoramic-type X-ray, either two-dimensional or three-dimensional. I use the more sophisticated 3D Cone Beam Scanner that produces images of your upper jaw, lower jaw, teeth and sinuses. It can't always detect early stages of bone death, but many lesions can be visualized on this type of X-ray. These scans are invaluable for the surgical planning aspect of treating these conditions.

Another diagnostic method that gives us clues is thermography, which has been used since the 1970s. Thermography and Thermometry (they are different) are now more commonly found in the offices of various types of healthcare practitioners and health coaches. These devices measure the temperature coming from the body.

There are two types of Thermogram devices. One utilizes an infrared camera to image the temperature of the part of the body in question. Most frequently used in the early diagnosis of breast cancer or some other temperature aberration such as that seen from a cavitation. The other type uses a point measurement system that captures specific temperatures being measured at points on the skin. The infrared camera data is read by a radiologist whereas the point measure is fed into a computer to compare and contrast your reading with that of an extensive data base.

Both are tools that help a practitioner peer into the body in a different manner. Recent advances in software and imaging technology have made these very useful techniques that let me see which areas of your skin are hotter than the surrounding area.

I also use an ultrasound imaging diagnostic method for detecting jaw bone lesions/cavitations. The ultrasound produces three-dimensional color graphs showing the bone's status with respect to moisture within the bone.

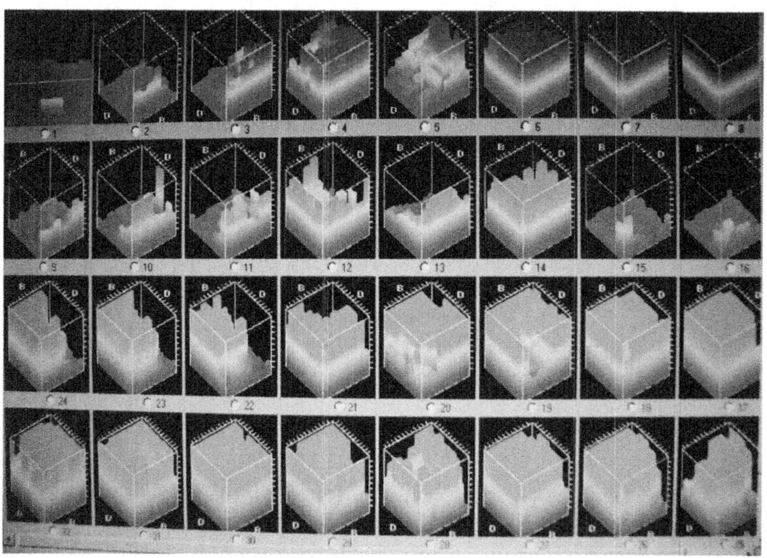

Image from my Cavitat® ultrasound

Mr. Bob Jones invented the FDA-approved Cavitat®, an ultrasound instrument designed to image jaw bones and detect cavitations. In his early research he scanned both males and females of various ages from several geographic areas of the United States.[12] He found cavitations of various sizes and severity under or near 94 percent of root canal filled teeth.

Another method I use to diagnose jaw bone cavitations are **diagnostic injections. This is a** relatively simple technique used to locate and confirm the presence of a cavitation. To do that, I inject a few drops of non-vasoconstrictive anesthetic into your gum tissue over a suspected site. After several minutes, a small hole is made into the bone with a tool, and approximately 1cc of the anesthetic is deposited into the body of the bone. We then wait a few additional minutes and evaluate the level of pain you are feeling. If my suspicion is accurate, you will have a dramatic reduction in your pain. By doing this one section or area after the other, I can gain a greater understanding of the relationship of the lesion to your well-being and the precise location of the lesion.

CASE STUDY

An 18-year-old male college student came to me with an emergency. His mother brought him to the Mayo Clinic in Arizona from St. Louis. His chief complaint was overwhelming fatigue. While at the Mayo Clinic, a whole battery of tests were done, but the doctors said they could find nothing wrong.

When I saw this young man, I took a detailed history and my preliminary diagnosis was a NICO lesion. I treated his upper jaw third molar sites with diagnostic blocks using anesthetic, and waited a few minutes. He had significant improvement in how he felt. I then administered the anesthetic to the lower jaw third molar sites. Within a few more minutes he felt 90 percent improvement in his overall well-being. His symptoms had begun while he was in school approximately 6 months after the removal of his wisdom teeth. X-rays appeared reasonably normal. Between his history and my awareness of these types of problems, I was able to accurately diagnose the problem and treat him by having the affected areas removed, resulting in a permanent cure.

Safe Treatment

You can get relief through the surgical treatment of cavitations. Holistic dentists agree with traditional practitioners, such as the renowned Dr. Black, that necrotic bone should be removed. However, there is a great divide within the profession as to the recognition of this condition and thus treatment.

The usual treatment of cavitations is to surgically debride (scrape clean the area), removing all of the unhealthy bone and pathology such as abscesses, cysts, etc. I don't recommend just "draining the lesion," nor do I advocate injecting homeopathic remedies alone into the lesion as the sole treatment nor other substances (except ozone) into the lesion because it may increase the severity of the damaged tissue. The notable exception is ozone.

After removing the unhealthy and dead (necrotic) bone, the next goal is to help regenerate the bone. Successful bone regeneration relies on your healing ability as well as the elimination of known risk factors. Risk factor elimination is not always possible but one strives to minimize the risk factors.

If you have faulty or incomplete healing, the lesion often returns and you will need to be treated again. No matter how well the surgery is performed you may experience this faulty healing if you have internal conditions that are ongoing. There are very few dentists who are trained to effectively diagnose and treat these lesions. Those who are not trained are really not qualified to diagnose this condition. The doctor, because of personal belief, may confidently assure you that you do not have any cavitations at all, when in reality you do. You then join the medical merry-go-round of the walking wounded who continue seek answers to their malady.

After the removal of the necrotic bone, the surgical site is irrigated and treated with various solutions to aid in the removal of bacteria and toxins, thereby decontaminating the site. If there is extensive bone damage, a bone regenerative material and/or absorbable membrane to guide new bone growth may be placed. To further assist with bone regeneration, platelet rich plasma and platelet rich fibrin alone or along with bone regenerative material can be placed in the surgical site to front load the site with growth factors and the body's own stem cells. The area is closed (sutured) with special sutures that help prevent bacterial reinfection.

Along with surgery, I also use both low-level and high-energy lasers to treat cavitations. These are two very different kind of lasers.

Low level laser therapy (LLLT) is used after a procedure has been performed. These low level lasers are applied to your skin and the energy is allowed to bathe the area that has just had the surgery. The frequency of light (860nm) emitted by the diodes was specially chosen because of its healing effects on tissues.[13] This creates a great deal of bio-stimulation that re-energizes the area, including the mitochondria that live inside your cells, giving you an enhanced ability to heal.

I use the FDA-approved Anodyne® unit to give patients low-level laser therapy. This is accomplished by placing pads containing special light emitting diodes, (LEDs) on the affected areas and other selected sites. It energizes the circulating blood thereby carrying the energy to your tissues where a substance called nitric oxide (NO) is produced. Nitric oxide is a very small, body-friendly molecule composed of single atoms of nitrogen and oxygen. It acts as a mediator in your system.

The benefit of NO is that it can relax smooth muscle tissue, dilate your lymphatic tissue, increase collagen production, reduce swelling and it's an anti-bacterial agent.

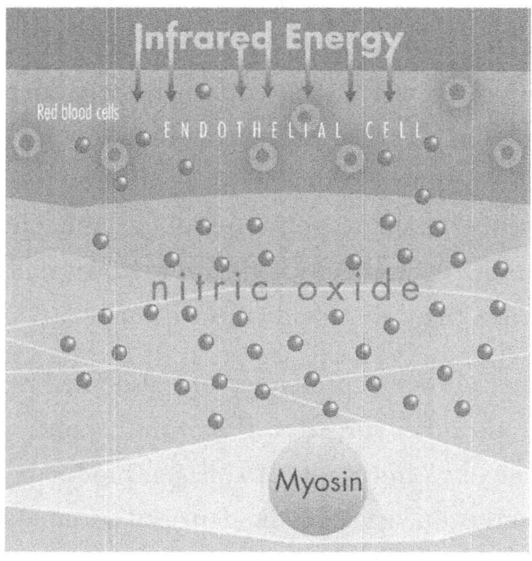

Nitric oxide (NO) is beneficial to your tissues

I also use a high-energy Neodymium Yttrium Aluminum Garnet (Nd:YAG) laser to denature the pathologic proteins and bacteria in the surgical site and to help cause a thermally initiated blood clot to form. A very simple example of denaturing a protein is what happens to an egg when it is cooked. The white goes from a clear gooey fluid to a white and firm substance. This laser is also used to remove the potential for pain from the needle stick sites. This is an amazing accessory in the management of post-operative pain.

Another way that can help encourage bone healing is through Hyperbaric Oxygen Therapy (HBOT). This therapy is best known for treating "the bends" that scuba divers can get if they rise too quickly underwater and bubbles of nitrogen form in their blood. HBOT forces oxygen into your cells, increasing the oxygen tension inside your damaged oxygen-depleted tissue. By providing more oxygen, it kills the bacteria that can't live on oxygen, and it improves circulation in the area and allows new bone or vascular tissues to grow and fill into the injured space. I do not have the equipment for this in my own office but there are local offices that can provide this treatment.

Oxidative Medicine principles are also used when I treat cavitations and other surgeries. Prolozone® is one such therapy. Treatment involves injections of collagen-producing substances, nutrients, and ozone gas into the damaged tissue in and around your joints.[14] It can dramatically lessen the pain as it helps the ligaments repair themselves.

Homeopathic remedies are also used in conjunction with other therapies to treat cavitations. I recommend homeopathic remedies not only for support for the cavitation surgery but for a variety of other surgeries in your mouth and elsewhere. Homeopathic therapies are versatile. I use them to open lymphatic drainage, support your liver for detoxification purposes, give you an overall general body healing and well-being, and support new bone growth and soft tissue healing. I use these homeopathic remedies as well as mainstream medicine and physical interventions in your treatment. As previously stated, I am not an advocate of using them, by themselves, for injection into a cavitation lesion.

There are several products, including enzymes, natural antimicrobials and healing nutrients that can give you nutritional and systemic support prior to and after the surgery. In some cases, limited antibiotics may be needed. It is important that all body detoxification pathways are open and functioning well: bowels, kidneys, skin, lungs, and especially the lymphatic system. Your electrolyte balance is also important for efficient detoxification and healing.

Intravenous Vitamin C (IV-C) can also assist with healing by helping to clean up the toxic materials and bacteria released into your bloodstream. This is considered an oxidative therapy. It is very safe and very effective.

TESTIMONY BY B.D.P

Now that I have completed all my dental work, I wanted to thank you for the outstanding care that you provided. Although the work was extensive, I had an extraordinary outcome and am very thankful for everything you did along the way. Your staff is amazing! I have never been in such a friendly dental office. Rhonda was so helpful during my first phone call to your office. She patiently answered all my questions and provided me with excellent information on what to expect during my consultation. This was especially important to me as I was experiencing significant health issues at the time. Jen was incredibly knowledgeable and genuinely kind person.

Thanks to your wisdom and experience, I am no longer suffering the ill effects of my previous dental problems. I am back at work full time and feeling great. You literally gave me my life back! Again, I wanted to let you know that I appreciate all you and your staff have done for me.

Prevention of Cavitations

Unfortunately there are few things you can do to help prevent cavitations from forming in your jaw. Since jaw bone cavitations are often found in the third molar area where your wisdom teeth live and may have been previously extracted, we have to keep a careful eye on that area. It is particularly susceptible because the tissue contains small terminal blood vessels that can cause bone death. You need to get your doctors on board here.

If you were "lucky" and didn't get one or more of your third molars, you have to ask the question why. Since the tooth didn't calcify it will not reveal itself on an X-ray. I can tell you with certainty, upon surgical debridement of these types of areas; I have yet to have one that would have been considered healthy from a microscopic perspective.

One way I can help prevent cavitations is by using a non-vasoconstricting (blood vessel constricting) anesthetic almost 99 percent of the time for dental procedures. Most dentists commonly use local anesthetics containing a vasoconstrictor (such as epinephrine), that reduces the blood flow and thus the oxygen supply to the bone in these areas. You don't want to do that because you could trigger destruction of the tissue in that area.

You can minimize your other risk factors by avoiding tooth extractions, periodontal surgery, root canal procedures (removing the alive or dead nervous tissue and intentionally leaving a dead tooth in the jaw), bruxism (tooth grinding), electrical trauma, metallic restorations (fillings such as mercury), galvanism (electric currents produced from mixed metals), high speed cutting (drilling), bacterial trauma (infections) and periodontal disease (biofilm disease). If you get therapy to treat these conditions, you are much more likely to suffer from jaw bone cavitations. Note that many of these things are done in the common course of dental care.

Your risk from cavitations can be reduced when your dentist correctly removes all of the dead, damaged, or infected tissue to improve the healing potential of the remaining healthy tissue after pulling your tooth (known as debridement). It is also helpful for your dentist to use new technologies, instruments, products, and technological applications for enhancing the bone regeneration process.

You may also have to make certain decisions when you're undergoing cancer treatment. Unfortunately studies have found that chemotherapy can cause osteonecrosis. In one study, all of the patients who had received treatment for their malignant bone disease with bisphosphonates had jaw bone cavitations.[15]

Conclusion

Holistic dentistry helps your overall health in a way that traditional dentistry does not when it comes to the treatment of jaw bone cavitations and root canals. That's because holistic dentists are very much aware of the relationship between the diseases in your body and the health of your teeth. I find the biggest obstacle to many of these types of ideas and treatments is simply the way that we are trained by conventional medical and dental perspectives, which are very narrow indeed.

End Notes

[1] "What Is Mitochondrial Disease?" *What Is Mitochondrial Disease - The United Mitochondrial Disease Foundation*. Web. 26 Feb. 2016.

[2] "Root Canal Dangers - Weston A Price." *Weston A Price*. 2010. Web. 26 Feb. 2016.

[3] Kokkas, A. B., A. Goulas, K. Varsamidis, V. Mirtsou, and D. Tziafas. "Irreversible but Not Reversible Pulpitis Is Associated with Up-regulation

of Tumour Necrosis Factor-alpha Gene Expression in Human Pulp." *International Endodontic Journal Int Endod J* 40.3 (2007): 198-203.

[4] Steinman, R.R., and J. Leonora. "Relationship of fluid transport through the dentin to the incidence of dental caries," Journal of Dental Research 50.6 (November 1971): 1536-1543.

[5] "Revolution Health Center." *Revyourhealth*. Web. 26 Feb. 2016.

[6] "About Paracelsus, A Holistic Healthcare Center." *About Paracelsus, A Holistic Healthcare Center*. Web. 26 Feb. 2016.

[7] AAE Position Statement. "NICO Lesions Neuralgia-Inducing Cavitational Osteonecrosis." *Endodontists: The Root Canal Specialists*. 2012. Web. 26 Feb. 2016.

[8] Bouquot, J. E. "Black's Forgotten Disease: NICO (neuralgia-inducing Cavitational Osteonecrosis)." *The Maxillofacial Center* (1994).

[9] Daunderer, Max. "Clinical Toxicology in Dentistry." *Ecomed* 1.3 (1995).

[10] Levy, T. E., and H. A. Huggins. "Routine Dental Extractions Routinely Produce Cavitations." *Journal of Advancement in Medicine* 9.4 (Winter 1996).

[11] Lechner, Johann, and Volker von Baehr. "RANTES and fibroblast growth factor 2 in jaw bone cavitations: triggers for systemic disease?" *Int J Gen Med.* 6 (2013): 277–290.

[12] "Patent US6030221 - Ultrasonic Apparatus and for Precisely Locating Cavitations within Jaw bones and the like." *Google Books*. Web. 26 Feb. 2016.

[13] Cobb, Charles M. "Lasers in Periodontics: A Review of the Literature." *Journal of Periodontology* 77.4 (2006): 545-64.

[14] Elvis, Am, and Js Ekta. "Ozone Therapy: A Clinical Review." *Journal of Natural Science, Biology and Medicine J Nat Sc Biol Med* 2.1 (2011): 66-70.

[15] Bagan, J. V., J. Murillo, Y. Jimenez, R. Poveda, M. A. Milian, J. M. Sanchis, F. J. Silvestre, and C. Scully. "Avascular Jaw Osteonecrosis in Association with Cancer Chemotherapy: Series of 10 Cases." *J Oral Pathol Med Journal of Oral Pathology and Medicine* 34.2 (2005): 120-23.

CHAPTER 6

BEWARE THE BIOFILM: PERIODONTAL DISEASE, LYME DISEASE & MARCONS

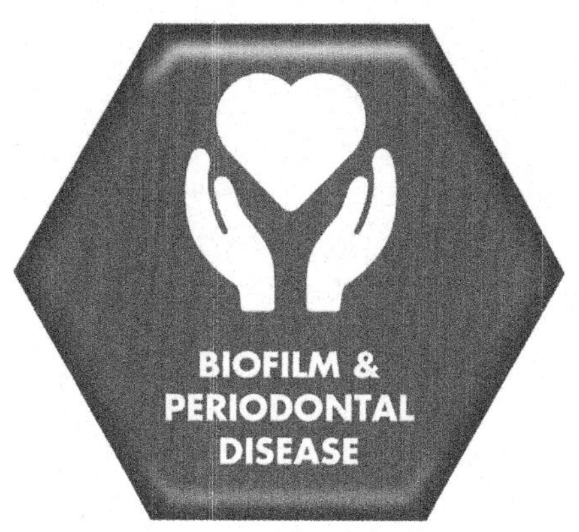

When you consult my Holistic Dental Matrix™, the most obvious signs of periodontal (gum) disease can be found in your teeth and gums. To understand periodontal disease, you have to be aware of the complex structures that make up your teeth. Periodontal disease, otherwise known as periodontitis, is a chronic inflammation of the periodontium, the connective tissue that surrounds the root of your tooth and attaches it to its bony socket. This periodontium is made up of fibers that extend into the bone as well as the different tissues that surround and support your teeth.

Typically, your gums shrink back from around the neck or base of the tooth, and your teeth become loose. You might see blood or pus at the neck of your teeth where it emerges from the gum, and you may be experiencing tooth pain or you are grinding your teeth.

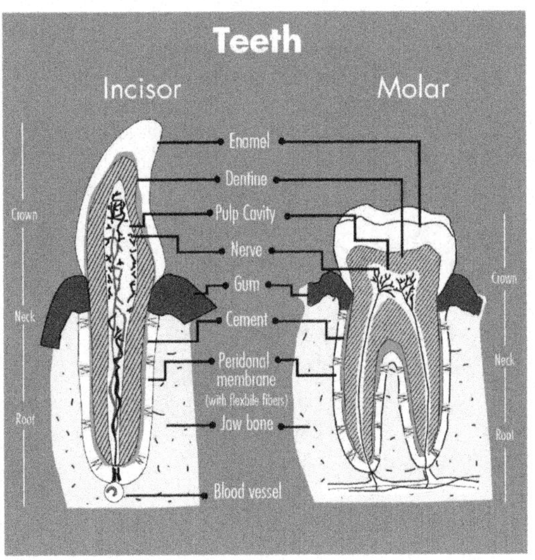

The complex anatomy of your teeth

However there are also a number of symptoms caused by periodontal disease that don't involve your teeth and gums. That's because the troubling signs of this disease can appear elsewhere in your body.

For example, you may have found your way to this chapter because you were diagnosed with lung cancer or pancreatic cancer. Or you may have given birth to a pre-term or low birth weight baby. Or you may be diabetic and find that you have insulin resistance, or suffer from coronary artery disease.

These kinds of symptoms can all be caused by periodontal disease. You have to treat periodontal disease aggressively when you see signs of it elsewhere in your body, because these visible signs show that the disease has progressed to the point where your whole system is breaking down.

Periodontal Disease

The tissues in your mouth get inflamed because of bacterial plaque on your teeth. Gingivitis is a mild form of periodontal disease that is caused by not brushing, flossing or water picking your teeth on a regular basis. With gingivitis, the soft tissues of your gums get irritated, redness and swelling occurs, and it can cause bad breath but the bone is untouched.

With the more advanced periodontal disease, all tissues are adversely impacted. There is destruction of your "alveolar bone," this is the part of jaw bone that holds the teeth in. It also affects your periodontal ligament, the connective tissue fibers that attach your tooth to the alveolar bone that it sits in.[1]

When you have periodontal disease, the epithelial (pink tissue) attachment, which connects to the tooth, can be affected. As the process of destruction advances, it moves in the direction of the root tips of your teeth. The outer layer of gum can stay high but the inner aspect is what suffers. This results in the formation of periodontal pockets, and the loosening of teeth and ultimately the loss of your teeth.

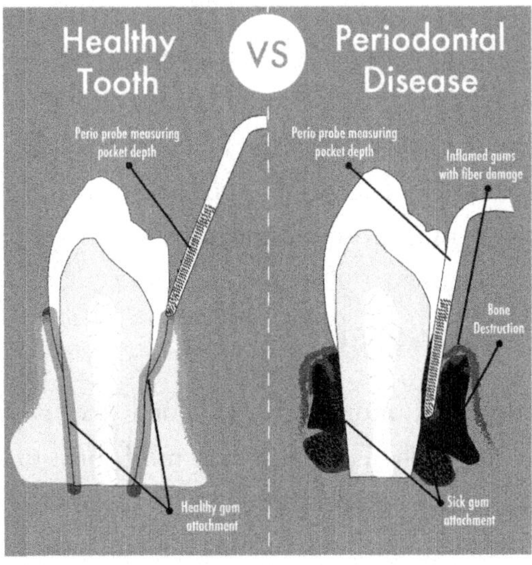

Diagnosing periodontal disease using a periodontal probe

To evaluate the extent of the damage, your dentist or hygienist will measure the depth of your gum attachment using a periodontal probe which is slipped between your tooth and gum.

Causes of Periodontal Disease

Periodontal disease is an infection of the gums that affects almost half of the adult population in the U.S. in some form or another. A study titled "Prevalence of Periodontitis in Adults in the United States: 2009 and 2010" estimates that 47 percent (64 million

American adults) have mild, moderate or severe periodontitis. In adults 65 and older, that rate increases to 70 percent.[2]

Periodontal disease, in part, starts with plaque, a sticky substance that forms on your teeth. Plaque is considered a biofilm. I'm sure you're thinking, "What is a biofilm?"

A biofilm is a bacterial slime that grows and grows over time, like a monster movie happening in your mouth. In fact, you can go to www.DrNicholasMeyer.com to see a real time movie of the development of a biofilm.

If you have ever seen the inside of a pipe when it has been taken off your kitchen sink, you probably found it slimy inside. That is also a biofilm.

This slime is a very organized environment of various life forms that include bacteria as well as proteins. If left undisturbed, the biofilm produced by the bacteria and other organisms, becomes a highly-functioning, self-organizing colony. They extract iron from blood cells, thus bursting the cells and can lead to anemia by a decrease in the red blood cells. You may not realize it, but bacteria are living organisms, just like a plant or human being. This means bacteria consume materials, release energy from food, release wastes, grow, respond to the environment and reproduce.

Bacteria are dependent on the pH of the area they live in, and they like to hide in undisturbed places. The outermost layer of this bacterial mix is aerobic while the deeper recesses of the mix can become anaerobic in nature. That means on the surface, the bacteria takes in oxygen to survive, but as the bacterial infection goes deeper and the oxygen is depleted, the organism changes to adapt. Once it becomes anaerobic, then the bacteria releases endotoxins which are harmful to the rest of your body.

One kind of biofilm illness to be aware of is nasal biofilms. They are thought to be "seeded" from the low grade infections found in teeth that have had root canal treatment and in dead teeth and jaw bone lesions (see Chapter 5 – Root Canal & Jaw Bone Lesions).

These nasal biofilms can contain MARCoNS (Multiple Antibiotic Resistant Coagulase Negative Staphylococci). This disease has been only recently identified and is somewhat similar to MRSA, the methicillin resistant staphylococcus aureus, except for what it does to a microbiological culture. Both are extremely difficult to eradicate from your body. MARCoNS has been found to reside in the inner deep recesses of the nose and in the tissue around teeth that have root canals. I have personally done microbiological assay confirmation of this phenomenon.

Furthermore, this kind of biofilm is often found in people who have Chronic Inflammatory Response Syndrome (CIRS) that has been found to be the result of mold. There are multiple symptoms characteristic of CIRS or mold toxicity. The symptoms show up after being exposed to mold (fungus) either in the home or in your place of work. Mold is not an innocuous life form.

The symptoms of CIRS are similar to some found in the Holistic Dental Matrix. These characteristics of CIRS have been compiled by Dr. Ritchie Shoemaker of Pokomoke, Maryland. Symptoms are: weakness, unusual pain, ice pick pain, cough, shortness of breath, joint pain, appetite swings, sweats (especially night sweats), temperature regulation problems, excessive thirst, increased urination and static shock. Further symptoms include: cognitive impairment, blurred vision, peripheral neuropathy and diarrhea or constipation.

Fighting Biofilm

In general, the only way to disturb dental biofilm (plaque) is to physically agitate it and break it loose. Biofilms are also sensitive to nanoparticle silver and also ozone gas. Doesn't that make you want to brush your teeth with good products?

As the biofilm accumulates on your teeth, if it isn't physically removed, it can start to harden or calcify. This happens as minerals come together to form what is known as tartar or calculus.

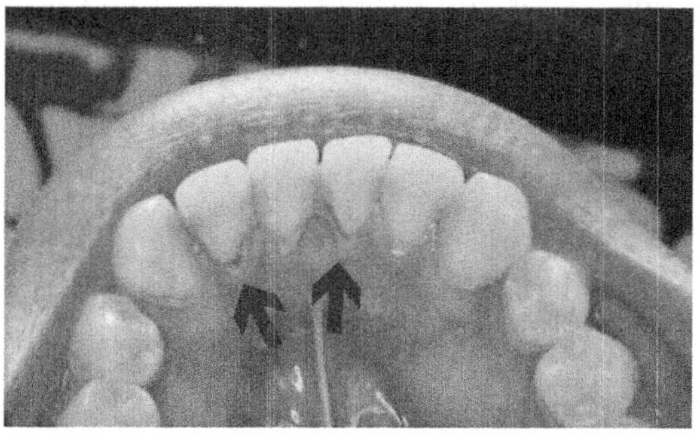

Tartar buildup on the inside of the lower front teeth

A curious thing is that in some people, the tartar seems to form in spite of good physical care. This phenomenon is dependent on the pH of the saliva and the surface energy of the tooth/teeth.

This tartar creates a rough surface that supports additional bacteria growth. As the bacteria grow, they further affect the soft tissue around your teeth. Symptoms of gingivitis include red swollen gums, bleeding, bad breath, and sometimes an unpleasant taste in your mouth.

This process of moving from plaque to gingivitis is affected by a number of factors, but not exclusively, like how healthy your immune system is. Do you eat plenty of fruits and vegetables, or do you eat processed food and sodas?

One example of how the food we eat can directly affect our teeth is scurvy. Scurvy is caused by a lack of Vitamin C in your diet. Your body needs Vitamin C to create collagen, which is the main part of connective tissue. It's that connective tissue that holds your teeth in your gums.

Back in the age of sail, people who took months-long ocean voyages weren't able to get fresh fruit and vegetables to eat. They didn't know it at the time, but this lack of Vitamin C caused their teeth to fall out. Scurvy put a damper on migration on a global level for hundreds of years, until researchers finally realized that fresh citrus could prevent scurvy. That's why the sailors from Britain way back in the day used to be referred to as "Limey" because they ate limes to ward off scurvy.

So the best way to prevent periodontal disease is to eat a balanced diet of nutritional food, get plenty of Vitamin C, and brush twice a day with baking soda or a special toothpaste. See www.DrNicholasMeyer.com for further info.

Untreated, gingivitis remains in a stable state of disease or it can worsen and become periodontitis, in which various bacteria and other life forms continue to grow and destroy both the gums and the supporting bone structures. Pockets can form where your teeth separate from the gums and surrounding bones. Left untreated, periodontitis eventually results in tooth loss.

Health Effects

Periodontal health is crucial to your overall health and well-being. As I've explained above, this disease involves many different tissues in your mouth. Those tissues are connected through direct pathways to other areas of your body, in the same way you've seen with TMD disorders and cavitations in Chapters 4 & 5.

It is not a new idea that periodontal health is connected with our overall health. It was first put forth in the mid-1920s by dental researcher Weston A. Price, D.D.S. Dr. Price stated that the bacteria that cause periodontal disease moves from the damaged tissues into root canal tissues and to other parts of your body.[3] His 10-year study of 14 tribal groups around the world concluded that traditional diets produce better physical health and emotional stability than a modern diet with processed food, sugars and milk-products.

This sort of disease migration through your body is well known with other kinds of illnesses, as well. When this occurs with cancer, it is known as metastasis. In a similar way, bacteria can metastasize from one place in your body to another place, seeding other diseases.

This happens because the bacteria in plaque activate your immune system to fight the inflammation. This triggers your body to release different proteins, like cytokines and heat shock proteins. Bacteria can even infect your blood, known as bacteremia, which is caused by the infection itself or because of dental treatments to repair the damage.[4]

Inflammation is a normal bodily process that is provoked by an injury. Generally, inflammation is a short-term process that brings the necessary elements together inside your body to repair injured tissue. That's how your body heals.

But there's a problem when inflammation is prolonged beyond the usual repair time. That happens when there's some kind of trickery or deception happening within your body that keeps the inflammation revved high. It can get stuck in the "on" position when there's really no need for it to be there.

One example of this is when you have a high filling. When a dentist puts a filling into your tooth, it is vitally important to get your "bite" correct. If the filling is left high, even in the micron range (.001") the sensitive ligament that holds the tooth in place can become inflamed and the tooth feels tender when you bite on it. If this is ignored, the tooth will continue to be sore for a very long time, perhaps even years.

Yet when the filling is filed down or adjusted, the pressure comes off the ligament and healing can take place. Unfortunately the longer the inflammatory process has gone on, the longer it takes to have the tooth return to comfort.

The same sort of process happens with periodontal disease. The chronic nature of the disease creates a perpetual, worsening cycle in your body. That's why chronic bacterial infections are linked with inflammatory markers in your blood such as C-Reactive Protein (CRP). C-Reactive Protein is one of the signs of heart disease, and has been shown to be a better predictor for heart disease than cholesterol levels.[5]

CRP is created in your liver to fight inflammation that occurs from any cause. Successful periodontal treatment can lower your CRP, and lowering your CRP decreases the risk of heart attack more than prescription drugs.[6] If your CRP reading is over 5 or if it does not decrease with periodontal treatment, it could indicate some other systemic infection, which should be followed up by your doctor.

This process is how chronic periodontal disease can play a role in the development of diseases like coronary artery disease (CAD)[7] and atherosclerosis, which is hardening of the arteries.[8] Strokes have also been found to be associated with on-going periodontal disease in older adults.[9]

If you have been diagnosed with cancer, you also need to consider whether periodontal disease may be playing a role. Research has found links between gum disease and oral cancer, upper GI and gastric cancers, lung cancer and esophageal cancer. One study by the Harvard School of Public Health (HSPH) and

Dana-Farber Cancer Institute found a significant association between periodontal disease and cancer of the pancreas.[10]

Another systemic disease that is associated with severe and progressive periodontal disease is diabetes. The inflammatory response is similar in diabetes and periodontal disease, both of which lead to poor healing and an increased susceptibility to infection.[11] Obesity and Type 2 diabetes are also associated with many metabolic disorders including insulin resistance, hypertension and atherosclerosis. Chronic inflammation, even when it's considered to be in the "healthy" range, has recently been declared part of the insulin resistance syndrome (metabolic disorders like diabetes) and can make metabolic disorders grow worse.[12]

Inflammation is even thought to be a factor in Alzheimer's disease, and studies have found that chronic periodontitis is associated with Alzheimer's disease.[13] That's because infection in your body can affect your central nervous system.

A link has also been found between periodontal disease and rheumatoid arthritis. In the third National Health and Nutrition Examination Survey of over 4,000 members of the general population, people with rheumatoid arthritis were more likely to have periodontal disease or a complete loss of their teeth.[14]

That's why I always suggest you take it seriously when you see signs of swollen, reddened or bleeding gums, because chronic periodontal disease can turn into much more serious problems that can destroy your health.

Safe Treatment

The good news is that periodontal disease is a treatable condition. The goal is to reduce your gum inflammation and thus bring down your C-Reactive Protein, leading to better overall health.

Traditional dentists want to help you keep your teeth, just like holistic dentists. The primary difference between the two is that the more traditional methods rely mostly on pharmaceutical drugs and aggressive surgical therapies while the holistic methods work to establish a better environment through the aid of ozone, lasers, micronutrients, lifestyle changes and "micro" surgery.

While traditional dentists recommend flap surgery to treat periodontal disease, I believe in the holistic dentistry solution of laser gum treatment, which is much less invasive than traditional surgery. Holistic treatments are kinder to the body and are therefore less painful than the more traditional method of surgery.

In 1999, I acquired the first laser in the nation that allowed dentists to use the patented procedure (LANAP). Later, in November 2005, I became a certified trainer with the Institute for Advanced Laser Dentistry teaching other doctors from around the country this wonderful procedure. Although I'm no longer actively training, I continue to research the inter-relationships of the factors involved in gum disease and your well-being.

In my experience, most patients prefer laser therapy over traditional surgery. The area of your mouth that is affected is treated with a local anesthetic before the treatment begins. And from there it's generally a comfortable experience.

Altogether, the benefits of laser treatment outweigh those of traditional periodontal flap surgery. First, it's much less painful and less traumatic on your body. You typically don't have to worry about bleeding, stitches or getting an infection because your gums haven't been cut wide open. Also, laser therapy is about 20 percent less expensive than traditional periodontal surgery, and it can be used to treat periodontal disease at almost any stage.

Even when you treat the diseased tissues, if the forces of your bite are not balanced correctly, the damage from the pressures remain and the treatment will have less than an optimal outcome and result in a short beneficial effect. That's why both issues need to be assessed and treated by laser therapy and bite therapy together for an effective solution.

The following are the steps involved in laser therapy:

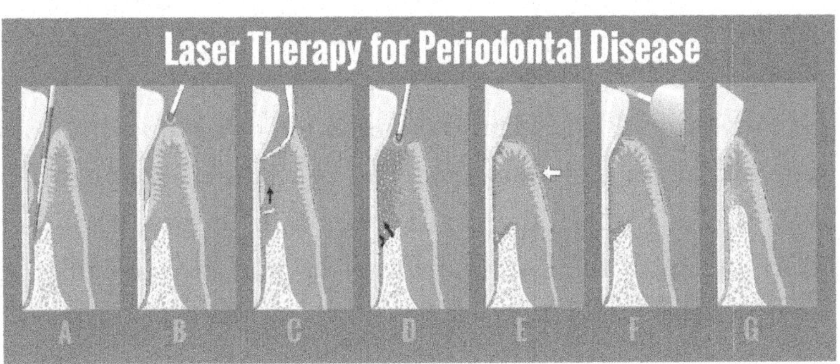

A. A periodontal probe measures to explore the defect between the tooth and gum.

B. Then I direct a small fiber optic cable between your tooth and gum that guides the laser energy at your gum tissues. Laser energy removes diseased tissues and denatures pathologic proteins. I can actually feel the roughness on your tooth through the fiber optic cable.

C. Next I use a combination of ultrasonic scalers with irrigants and hand instruments to cleanse the root surface of the contaminated layers.

D. Once a tooth is deemed to be clean, I use the laser to sterilize the pocket and cause a coagulum (blood clot) to form. It is within this coagulum, over time, that healing occurs and you form a new attachment between the bone and the tooth.

E. Then I use my finger to compress the gum tissues against the tooth. A stable fibrin clot forms at the crest of your gum.

F. Then, your bite is checked and if necessary, your tooth is filed down to prevent occlusal trauma, which is excessive pressure from opposing teeth.

G. Your healing is then monitored and you are seen for periodic maintenance visits. It is during these visits that ozone and/or laser energy are used for supplemental care.

Another treatment I've found to be beneficial on advanced periodontal disease is ozone infusion of the gum. Go here for explanatory video:

Our body runs on oxygen because it's a life-giving substance. That's why there are minimal side effects to ozone therapy, which has been studied for over a century in various countries. In 1979, Dr. George Freibott successfully used ozone to treat a Haitian AIDS patient suffering from Kaposi's sarcoma. Four years later, the first International Ozone Association medical ozone conference was held in Washington, D.C., resulting in a book called "Medical Applications of Ozone," compiled and edited by Julius Laraus.[15]

Ozone therapy is just one of a group of Oxidative Therapies, previously described, that have been found to be helpful in healing. Ozone is O^3, a potent gas that is antimicrobial, anti-fungal and anti-viral. By infusing medical grade ozone gas around your teeth and gums, I can treat the deepest of periodontal pockets.

The ozone is delivered in isolated areas via a small canula placed where desired or through specialized trays that have been custom made to conform to your mouth and teeth. It depends on what the desired outcome is. With the tray system there is an "in" port and "out" port that creates the free exchange of the gas. This is perfectly safe for your teeth and gums. If you happen to smell the ozone, then the flow can be altered to stop that.

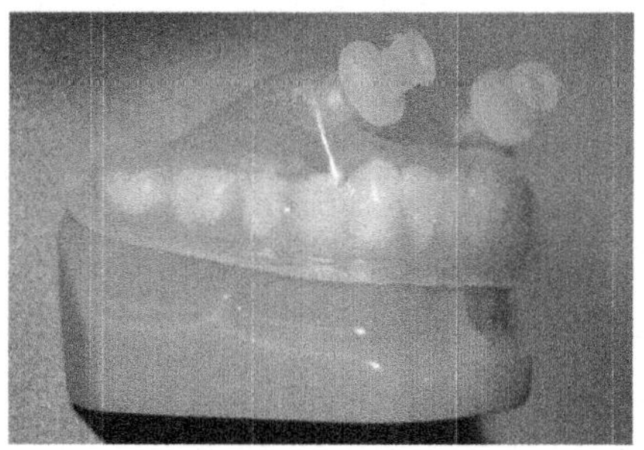

Ozone delivery tray

I also use ozone therapy to treat the previously mentioned bacterial biofilm infection, MARCoNS. The ozone is infused directly into the tissues of the upper jaw that are adjacent to the floor of the nose and sinuses. It has spurred study now into the relationship of the teeth to both MARCoNS and CIRS. Stay tuned for further developments on my website www.DrNicholasMeyer.com.

Along with laser and ozone therapy, sometimes additional treatments are needed to manage periodontal disease, including gum grafting and bone grafting using artificial, animal donor or tissue taken from elsewhere in your body.

I may also need to treat you with platelet-rich plasma (PRP) which is blood plasma that has been enriched with platelets. PRP contain growth factors, stem cells and cytokines that stimulate the healing of bone and tissue. This procedure can enhance a number of different dental therapies, not just periodontal disease.

Dental Implants

If the worst happens and periodontal disease is allowed to run its full course, then you will eventually lose the teeth that are affected. How and when that happens depends on your overall health and the strength of your bones. At that point, you have to decide if you're going to live without those teeth for the rest of your life.

There are various types of dental appliances that can be used to replace missing teeth. Some of these devices can be worn on the bone with no further support from your teeth. Other devices may take advantage of any remaining teeth for their support. Yet there can be a problem if your gums have been damaged by periodontal disease, because the teeth you have left are stressed and overworked even more by having to support the dental prosthesis.

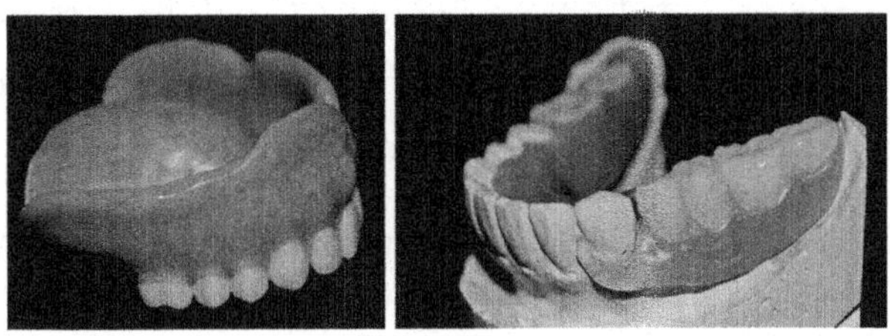

Full and partial dentures

For people who lose all of their teeth, a full denture is perhaps the only treatment option for them. This is a prosthetic device that carries all the teeth of the arch. However, this isn't always the best option because a complete denture has only approximately 25 percent of the effectiveness of your natural teeth.

A better option may be the use of dental implants. Simply stated, a dental implant is an artificial tooth root. They can take the form of simply a single tooth, small spans of multiple teeth or dental implants to support a complete dental prosthesis (full denture). The limiting factor here is how much available bone is present to place a dental implant. This also takes into account any vital structures such as nerves, arteries and sinuses that may influence the placement of a dental implant to carry a tooth or multiple teeth.

I use the latest advances in dental implants from Europe at Millennium Dental Associates as well as the traditional implants that are typically made from titanium, but now there are different types of materials that have become popular with both patients and holistic dentists. I discuss implant materials and their effect on your body in more depth in Chapter 2 – Heavy Metal… And Not the Rock Band Kind!

There are benefits to using non-metal implants, including the fact that it can help prevent bone deterioration that can occur over time. Also you can chew food normally because the tooth feels the same as your natural teeth and it blends well with the rest of your teeth. The biggest reason is a reduced risk of allergy or sensitivity issues, because some people are sensitive to metal.

I also use non-metal implants because I'm concerned about "oral galvanism," which is the electrical current that can happen in your mouth when metal restorative materials are used. This negative health effect happens because the saliva in your mouth connects all of the metal pieces. In the long run, non-metal implants are safer.

Non-metal implants are typically created using zirconium dioxide (ZrO_2), more commonly referred to as Zirconia, which is a ceramic material. One of the biggest advantages to this material is the fact that it has a natural white color instead of the silver color of titanium. Zirconia has been shown to be comparable to titanium in clinical longevity, since it does not easily corrode.

Zirconia dental implants also aren't as sensitive to temperature changes, like metal is, so you can't feel the same discomfort from hot or cold foods. It's also resistant to the natural acids that are created in your mouth for digestion, and to some of the cements that are used to retain the crowns (the artificial upper part of a tooth visible in the mouth).

Dental implants can vary depending on how they are placed in your mouth. There are "endosteal" implants that are placed *into* the bone, as well as "subperiosteal" which are implants that are placed *onto* the bone. Endosteal implants are the most common, and they are placed in your jaw bone by drilling a small hole into the bone and then an implant is screwed in place.

The process of getting a functional implant is a long one, typically taking up to 3 to 8 months to complete. That's because we have to start by placing the implant under your gums where it remains for 3 to 6 months. During this waiting period, your jaw bone bonds biologically to the implant, and a temporary bridge or denture is often used for cosmetics and space maintenance. Usually a soft diet is prescribed for the first few weeks.

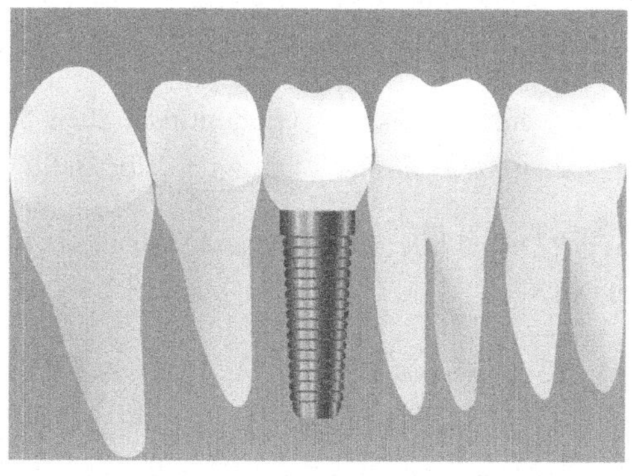

The implant screw is embedded in your jaw, and then the tooth is attached on top

After 3 to 6 months, your gums are opened up to uncover the implant and a post is attached. Two to 6 weeks later, the treatment is finished when the replacement tooth is fitted into the implant in your mouth.

Conclusion

The goal of holistic dentistry is to save your teeth and treat your gums so that periodontal disease doesn't ruin your health by provoking inflammation elsewhere in your body. As you can see from the information in this chapter, keeping your teeth and gums clean can help prevent a host of systemic diseases, whereas letting periodontal disease spread can worsen your condition. Since periodontal disease is very treatable, you owe it to yourself to take care of it now.

End Notes

[1] Kinane, Denis F. "Causation and pathogenesis of periodontal disease." *Periodontology* 25.1 (Feb. 2001): 8–20.

[2] Papapanou, P.N. "The Prevalence of Periodontitis in the US:Forget What You Were Told." *Journal of Dent. Res.* 91 (Aug. 30, 2012): 907-908.

[3] Price, Weston A. "Dental Infections Oral and Systemic." Oral Health 13.12 (Dec. 1923).

[4] Bartova, Jirina, P. Sommerova, Y. Lyuya-Mi, J. Mysak, J. Prochazkova, J. Duskova, T. Janatova, and S. Podzimek. "Periodontitis as a Risk Factor of Atherosclerosis." *Journal of Immunology Research* 2014 (2014): 1-9.

[5] Ridker, P.m, M.j Stampfer, and N. Rifai. "Novel Risk Factors for Systemic Atherosclerosis. A Comparison of C-reactive Protein, Fibrinogen, Homocysteine, Lipoprotein (a), and Standard Cholesterol Screening as Predictors of Peripheral Arterial Disease." *ACC Current Journal Review* 10.5 (2001): 25-26.

[6] Betteridge, D. John, J. Martin Gibson, and Philip T. Sager. "Comparison of Effectiveness of Rosuvastatin Versus Atorvastatin on the Achievement of Combined C-Reactive Protein." *The American Journal of Cardiology* 100.8 (2007): 1245-248.

[7] Geerts, Sabine O., Victor Legrand, Joseph Charpentier, Adelin Albert, and Eric H. Rompen. "Further Evidence of the Association Between Periodontal Conditions and Coronary Artery Disease." *Journal of Periodontology* 75.9 (2004): 1274-280.

[8] Scannapieco, Frank A., Renee B. Bush, and Susanna Paju. "Associations Between Periodontal Disease and Risk for Atherosclerosis, Cardiovascular Disease, and Stroke. A Systematic Review." *Annals of Periodontology* 8.1 (2003): 38-53.

[9] Lee, Hyo-Jung, Raul I. Garcia, Sok-Ja Janket, Judith A. Jones, Ana Karina Mascarenhas, Thayer E. Scott, and Martha E. Nunn. "The Association Between Cumulative Periodontal Disease and Stroke History in Older Adults." *Journal of Periodontology* 77.10 (2006): 1744-754.

[10] Michaud, D. S., K. Joshipura, E. Giovannucci, and C. S. Fuchs. "A Prospective Study of Periodontal Disease and Pancreatic Cancer in US Male Health Professionals." *JNCI Journal of the National Cancer Institute* 99.2 (2007): 171-75.

[11] Schmidt, Maria Inês, Bruce B. Duncan, A. Richey Sharrett, Gunnar Lindberg, Peter J. Savage, Steven Offenbacher, Maria Inês Azambuja, Russell P. Tracy, and Gerardo Heiss. "Markers of Inflammation and Prediction of Diabetes Mellitus in Adults (Atherosclerosis Risk in Communities Study): A Cohort Study." *The Lancet* 353.9165 (1999): 1649-652.

[12] Nishimura, F., Y. Soga, Y. Iwamoto, C. Kudo, and Y. Murayama. "Periodontal disease as part of the insulin resistance syndrome in diabetic patients." *J Int Acad Periodontol* 7 (2005): 16-20.

[13] Kamer, Angela R., Ronald G. Craig, Ananda P. Dasanayake, Miroslaw Brys, Lidia Glodzik-Sobanska, and Mony J. De Leon. "Inflammation and Alzheimer's Disease: Possible Role of Periodontal Diseases." *Alzheimer's & Dementia* 4.4 (2008): 242-50.

[14] de Pablo, P., et al. "Association of periodontal disease and tooth loss with rheumatoid arthritis in the US population." *The Journal of Rheumatology* 35.1 (2008): 70-76.

[15] Kramer, Fritz. "Ozone in the Dental Practice." *Medical Applications of Ozone.* Julius Laraus (ed.) Norwalk, CT: International Ozone Association, Pan American Committee. (1983): 258-65.

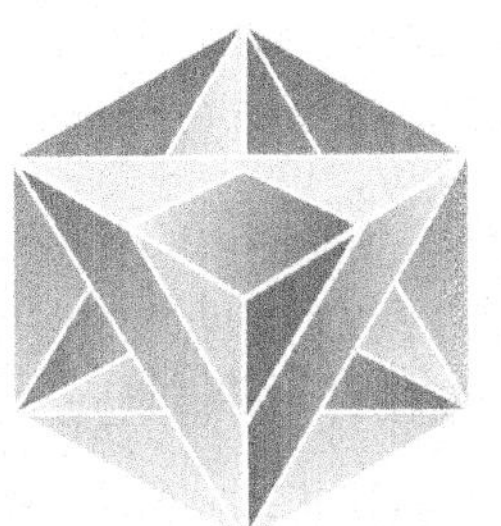

CHAPTER 7

HOLISTIC DENTAL DIAGNOSTICS AND TESTING: GETTING TO THE ROOT OF THE PROBLEM

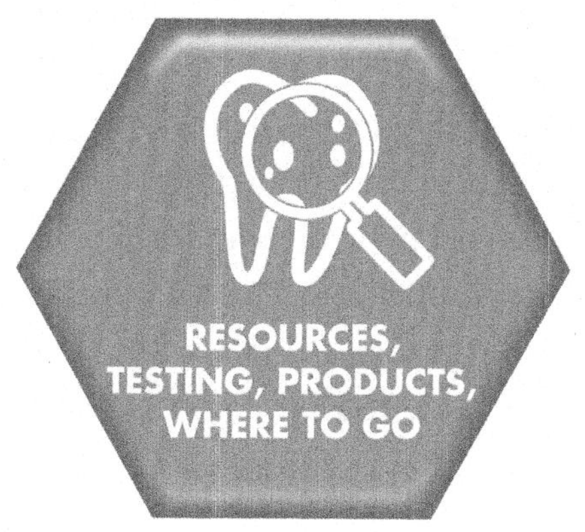

In this chapter, I bring together the various testing and diagnostic methods that holistic dentists use to determine the state of your health. You may have been to a number of different dentists throughout your life, but you may never have been offered these tests before. That's because many dentists stay in the comfort zone of the knowledge base that they acquired while they studied in the hallowed halls of academia and they don't venture too far out from that basic skill set.

One of the main reasons for this is because of the quality and quantity of continuing education that is required by the regulatory boards that govern the dental profession in each state. All medical professionals need to get ongoing training and education in order to stay on top of the latest scientific advances. But they are somewhat limited by the laws that govern what is considered acceptable. It takes a bit of searching to find classes that would be considered outside the box. It's also not easy to find a willingness to implement new ideas that come from outside of the "recommended" avenues.

This may be unsettling news that dentists can maintain their license without necessarily improving their competency or better still, becoming a more accomplished practitioner through advanced training. In my state, the basic requirement is a total of 72 hours over a 3-year span and almost 20 of those hours are not in clinical dentistry. You can find the requirements of your own State on the American Dental Association's website: www.ada.org.

In my experience, dentists need training in a high-tech approach in order to diagnose the cause of your problems, while they also have to deliver your care in a high-touch manner. This means it's important to keep the human involvement, such as understanding each patient and listening to their story to find the links in the chain that can lead you to the source of their problems.

This idea was put forth thirty years ago by John Naisbitt who wrote about the importance of a balanced high-tech approach in the #1 *New York Times* bestseller: *Megatrends: Ten New Directions Transforming Our Lives.* More recently in his book, *High Tech High Touch: Technology and Our Search for Meaning,* Naisbitt examined how we can make the most of technology's benefits without losing the human touch.

I think that is an admirable philosophy for medical practitioners to follow and it is something I do in my own practice when I'm diagnosing and treating my patients.

To better help you understand what sort of care you need, I will attempt to bring to life the tests you can take to discover the root of your problems. It is up to your doctor to use their knowledge base to pull together meaningful information and understand the story of what is happening to you in order to get the complete picture.

Airway Problems

Airway problems from snoring to sleep apnea are discussed along with the health problems this disorder can cause in Chapter 4 – TMD and Airway Disorders: I Haven't Got Time for the Pain. Airway obstructions create a lack of oxygen in your body, which stresses your entire system and puts you into a constant fight or flight state.

Here, I'd like to go over the various diagnostic tests that I use to gain insights into what may be causing your airway disorders.

Acoustic Reflection

This includes Acoustic Reflection Rhinometry and Acoustic Reflection Pharyngometry. These two diagnostic tools are used to map the internal structures of your nose (Rhinometry) and your mouth and throat (Pharyngometry).

For this test, a sensor is placed up to your nostril and a sound wave is beamed into your nasal cavity. This wave travels through the open space until it hits bone, and then it bounces back. That reflection can be read by the computer. In the case of the Pharyngometer, a sensor is placed in the mouth and the sound wave is beamed into your mouth and throat.

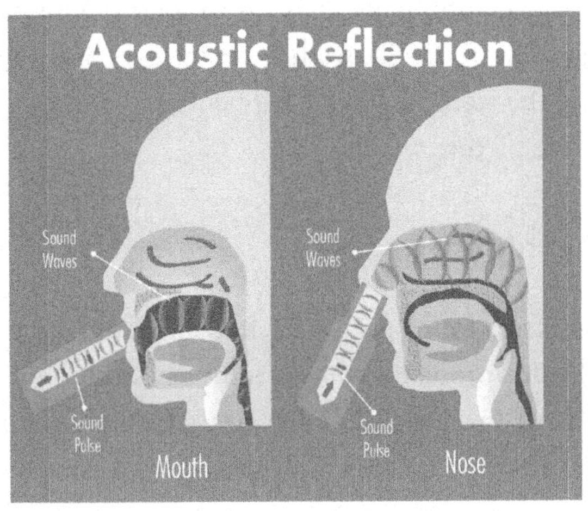

Diagnosing the size of the airway

The posture or position of your jaw can be altered to simulate any number of different jaw positions. The data reveals the changes in the volume of your mouth and throat. I can see where your airway needs to be opened up, and the best position for your jaw to accomplish that.

With this information, I can then make an educated decision to determine which oral device would work best for you. The best thing about acoustic reflection is that it's not an X-ray, so it doesn't expose you to radiation. Instead, it uses sound waves which aren't harmful. That means I can use it during your treatment to see how well your appliance is working, and to adjust it if needed.

3D Radiography

Also known in dentistry as Cone Beam Computed Tomography (CBCT), this diagnostic tool is indispensable in my practice. This X-ray includes your teeth, jaws, airways and jaw joints. It's a superb method of capturing the interior structure of your head and neck to see your airway issues.

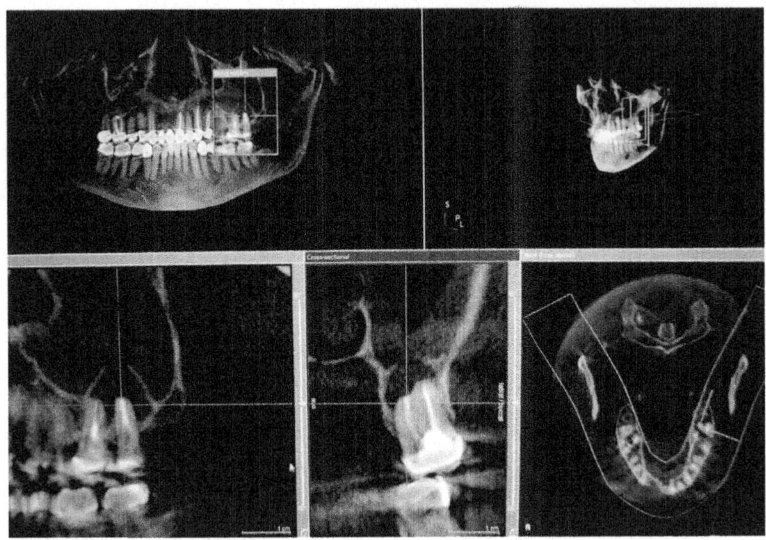

Images from a CBCT scan

One image can capture more data than you can imagine, allowing me to rapidly assess the various problem points. The ability to see your airway, TM joints, neck position, bone deformations, and bone and tooth pathology is almost dizzying. I can watch your movement in action, to see how everything in your mouth, jaw and throat are working together simultaneously.

If you consult a doctor who is comfortable with this tool, you can get much more useful data than ever before and make better choices based on that information.

Cavitations and Root Canals

Cavitations are diseased areas in your jaw bone. One common cause of cavitations is a root canal, which can trap bacteria in your tooth. The bacteria then spread to the surrounding bone. Once a lesion forms in your jaw, it creates potent enzyme-inhibiting substances that travel around your body wreaking havoc. Other reasons you can get cavitations are poor circulation, and improper healing after extractions.

You can find more information on the root causes and health problems that are created by cavitations in Chapter 5 – Root Canals and Jaw Bone Lesions: Hidden Causes of Disease. To diagnose cavitations, I use the following tests:

3D Radiography

I suggest you only take cavity-detecting X-rays once every five years to minimize your radiation exposure. A better method is to use 3D radiography, which I discuss above in "Airway Problems."

Cone Beam Computed Tomography (CBCT) can detect many, but not all cavitations. One of the benefits is that you get 90 percent less radiation exposure compared with traditional CT X-rays. Since it is digital, that means it's safer for the environment due to the lack of chemicals needed for the X-ray processing. It is also much quicker for your doctor to read as a result of the almost instantaneous images that are generated.

Ultrasound Imaging

I use a medical grade ultrasound to help detect cavitations. Ultrasound is a non-invasive diagnostic procedure that uses high-frequency sound waves. When these waves pass through your body, the waves produce images of your boney structures and even your blood flow.

I use a Cavitat® machine to scan through your jaw bone, and the images are immediately reproduced on my computer monitor. I look for weaknesses in the bone to focus my diagnostic efforts.

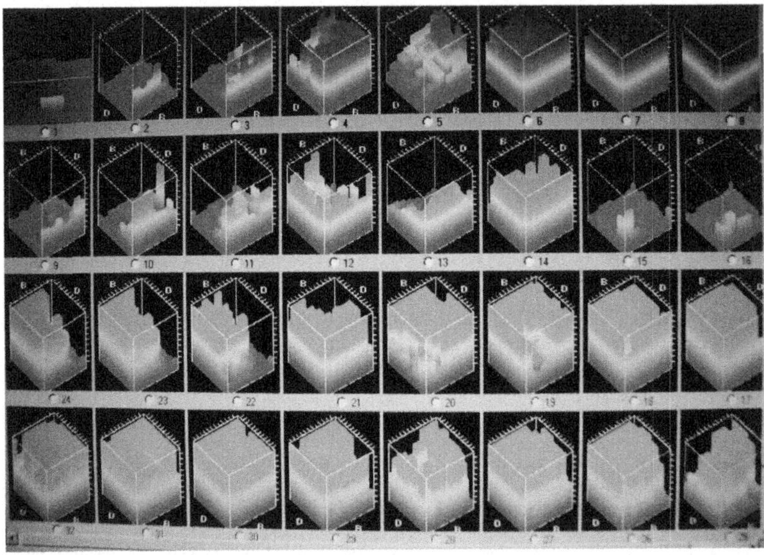

Images from my Cavitat® ultrasound

Thermography

Another diagnostic tool I use to discover cavitations is thermography. There are two forms of thermography: contact thermography or the more common infrared thermal imaging.

Both of these technologies test your body's ability to regulate heat that is under the control of your autonomic nervous system.

I look for irregularities within the patterns of heat images that can suggest some form of infection.

These tools are often used by health practitioners who find hot spots emanating from your head and neck area. These hot spots can be caused by a jaw bone cavitation, myofascial pain dysfunction syndrome, gum disease and other maladies.

Autonomic Response Testing

Autonomic Response Testing (ART) is a form of what is commonly referred to as muscle testing. The modern method is a derivation from standard orthopedic testing principles. A muscle is picked and tested to see how it locks a joint. It is not intended to be a test of strength but simply how a joint locks when loaded.

This sort of muscle monitoring is also called applied kinesiology (AK).[1] These kinds of tests are used for the development of rehabilitation programs for people with weak or damaged muscles. Each muscle can be checked to see if it tests weak or strong.

This form of testing is popular with many practitioners and is used in a variety of applications from physical health to emotional health.

Diagnostic Blocks

Another method I use to diagnose jaw bone cavitations are Diagnostic Blocks. This is a relatively simple technique in which I inject a tiny amount of non-vasoconstrictive anesthetic into your gum tissue over a suspected site that I've found using one of the methods above, such as CBCT, ultrasound or ART. Then I watch for a response, to see if the pain lessens. By doing this slowly one section after the other, I can gain a greater understanding of the condition and location of the source lesion.

Meridian Tooth Chart

When you're not suffering from any pain, the meridian tooth chart can help point me in the right direction. When a tooth or your jaw under a tooth becomes infected, your organs on the same acupuncture meridian can also become unhealthy. This energy flow goes both ways, so if you have a dysfunction in one of your organs, it can affect the corresponding tooth.

These meridians in our bodies have been stimulated through acupuncture and other Chinese healing practices for thousands of years. Your life force energy or "Qi" passes through these meridians. Some people believe this phenomenon is tied to the life force that flows through our past lives and future ones.

In the late 1940s, Dr. Reinhard Voll, a German doctor and engineer, created the diagnostic method of electroacupuncture. He documented the relation of changes in the energy to objective tests like blood tests.[2]

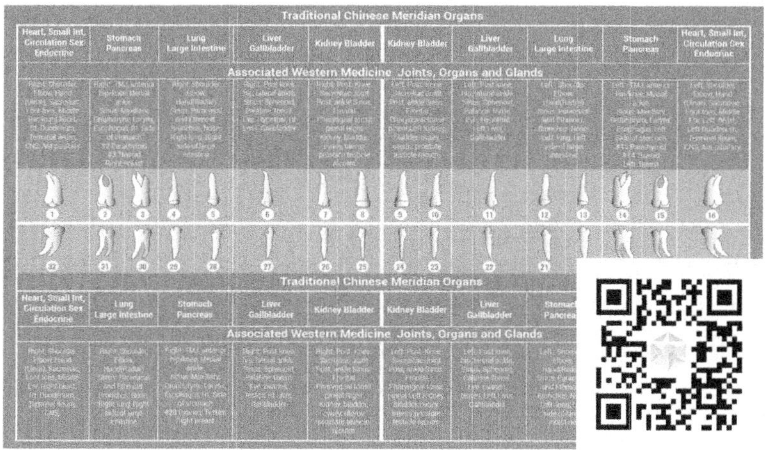

Meridian chart showing the relationship of each tooth to your organs, adaptation by Drs. Louisa Williams and Dietrich Klinghardt. An interactive chart is available on my website: follow QR code.

The Meridian Tooth Chart is based on traditional Chinese medicine and beliefs about the way your life-force flows through your body. The chart is said to have been developed by Thomas Rau, M.D., of the Paracelsus Clinic (Switzerland) and is based on work by Dr. Reinhard Voll and others.[3]

For example, if you're having stomach issues, it could be related to cavitations under your upper molars.

Dental Materials

Different kinds of dental materials are known to cause a wide range of health problems. I go into much more detail about metals and other kinds of dental materials, discussing the symptoms and reasons why these different materials can cause disease in Chapter 2 – Heavy Metal… And Not the Rock Band Kind! Here's a few of the tests I perform to detect which materials are affecting you in a negative way.

Oral Galvanism Testing

One very easy test to administer to see if metals are impacting you is through oral galvanism testing. This determines the level of the electric current in your mouth caused by the metals in your fillings, crowns and implants. Galvanism creates a measurable electric current of varying strength but I have measured about 120 millivolts in a patient's mouth, which is much higher than your body's usual 20 millivolts. If you have a high electrical current, then that can indicate the metals in your mouth are reacting against each other and overloading your nervous system with excess energy. This can result in the unexplained irritability and brain fog reported by sufferers.

Bio-energetic Resonance Testing

Another way I look to see if metals are affecting your body is by using diagnostic devices that test your bio-energetic resonance. This includes Autonomic Response Testing (ART), and computer-based resonance testing.

ART uses muscle biofeedback that lets me know if a muscle is weak when an interference (non-coherent) field is stimulated. It's an easy test to administer. I touch the probes to both points—your tooth and the problem area—to see if they are linked.

Another form of resonance testing I use is an ohmmeter to measure the electrical conductivity (resistance) of your skin at various acupuncture points. This technology is based the same principle used in lie detector and biofeedback devices. Common devices that measure electrical conductivity on the market are devices with names like: Biotron®, Dermatron®, Avatar®, Listen®, Zyto®, and others.

To conduct this kind of test, a probe is applied to various acupuncture points on your body and a tiny electrical current is sent through the circuit. These devices are very responsive so I can take a lot of readings to pinpoint what your conductivity value is for each area compared to the standards set by healthy people. Some units use a hand cradle to access this energy system.

Dental Materials Compatibility Test

For many patients, I suggest doing a Dental Materials Serum Compatibility Test to see how sensitive your body is to different dental materials. This includes not only metals but items such as bonding agents, impression materials, and the like.

To do this test, a small amount of blood is drawn from you. The sample is spun down in a centrifuge and the serum is then subsequently exposed to a variety of substances common to dental materials. This gives us a guide as to what materials are least reactive with your system as well as the ones that are the most reactive to your system that you want to avoid.

You can do this test yourself with a kit that is available through www.DrNicholasMeyer.com. You will get the results with an exhaustive list of thousands of dental materials that are screened specifically for your safety and immune challenges.

Also available through my website are kits that analyze your hair minerals to assess your body's load of metals and other harmful substances.

Fluoride

I discuss the harmful effects of fluoride in Chapter 3 – Fluoride: More Foe than Friend? The most visible sign of fluoride over-exposure is dental fluorosis, which is brown mottling on your teeth. But unfortunately, as of now, there is no specific test to check the fluoride burden in your body.

However there are tests you can do on your water to find out how much fluoride is in it. There's the easy and quick method, which uses fluoride detection test paper that you dip into the water. This detects even trace amounts of fluoride ions or hydrofluoric acid.

There are also EPA-rated tests for drinking water that use the SPADNS method, which involves putting water into a pre-packed ampoule with chemicals in order to see the results.[4]

Periodontal Disease

Health problems caused by periodontal disease are discussed in Chapter 6, along with the different kinds of bone and tissues that are involved.

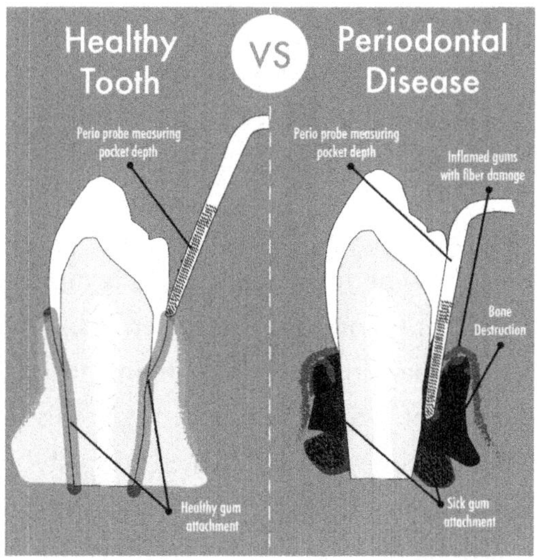

Healthy gums vs. Periodontal Disease

To diagnose periodontal disease, the traditional method is to use a periodontal probe to slip between your tooth and gum to see how deep the pocket is. X-rays can also be used to see the physical structures of your teeth.

Also available is a microbiology test called My Perio Path®. Here the doctor or hygienist samples the fluids from the mouth and sends it for analysis to see what kind of bacterial load you have in your mouth.

Blood Tests

There are other tests that can detect the bacterial infections that cause periodontal disease, such as a blood test. This can show you if you have inflammatory markers including C-Reactive Protein

(CPR). CRP is created in your liver to fight inflammation that occurs from any cause. If your CRP reading is high (+5), then successful periodontal treatment may lower it.

DNA Probe Test

The DNA probe test can identify the bacteria causing the disease so that the right antibiotic can be prescribed. More than 350 unique species of bacteria have been found to exist in plaque samples taken from periodontal patients.[5] This DNA probe test can be done before you are treated to establish a baseline. Then you have treatments as necessary to reduce the bacterial load. It can also be done after your treatment to ascertain the effectiveness of the treatment and your home care.

Bio-Energetic Feedback

Bio feedback can be a very helpful informational tool that detects energy through acupuncture meridian pathways. I also use these kinds of tests in diagnosing cavitations and problems with dental materials. There are a number of different types of bio-feedback analyses available to us.

Through computerized analysis of bio-energetic feedback, I can see the signs of toxins, bacteria and other pathogens that may be present. You take this test by touching a diagnostic machine that sends a signal along your skin to somewhere else in your body. Upon receiving the signal, your body responds. That response is recorded and analyzed with the data displayed on a screen. Applied kinesiology and Autonomic Response Technique are manual methods of assessing the energetic shifts of the system when challenged.

TMD

In Chapter 4 – TMD and Airway Disorders: I Haven't Got Time for the Pain, I discuss the wide variety of ailments that can come from having a bad bite, including chronic pain and systemic diseases. Here, I'll go into greater detail about the way I diagnose these kinds of TMD problems.

Often signs of TMD are immediately visible because of flat spots on your teeth or notches in the enamel at the base of your gum line from grinding your teeth. TMD can also be detected from the tenderness in the muscles in your jaw, and the amount of movement your jaw has. But to find out exactly what is going wrong with your bite so it can be fixed, you'll need to experience some diagnostic methods that were specially designed to uncover TMD.

Digital Biomedical Testing

I use electromyography to measure the muscle activity of your jaw muscles. This is done through surface electrode technology. You are probably more familiar with an EKG to diagnose heart problems, with electrodes placed on your chest to pick up the electrical signal of your heartbeats.

Technology today enables us to capture signals from skeletal muscles beneath the skin and display these signals on a computer monitor. By placing the patches (electrodes) on your skin we can evaluate in a real time manner how you are working or not working. Holistic dentists are interested in the muscles as a functional unit. One question that needs to be answered in this way is: How functional are the muscles and what is keeping them from maximal function?

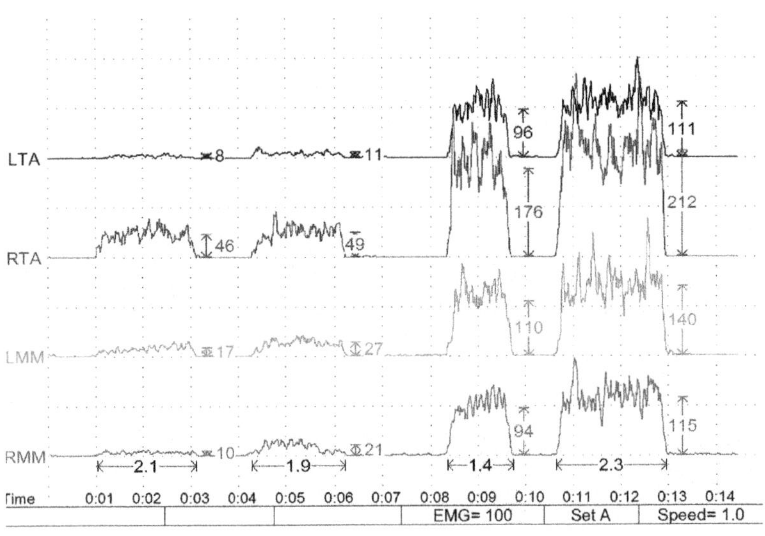

Units of energy are expressed in microvolts

The magic of this diagnostic tool can be seen when we challenge the muscle to perform and we see how it functions. Take a look at this example below of a readout which shows four "bursts" of energy. In this example, you are looking at two paired muscle groups: the right and left temple muscles (LTA & RTA) and the right and left chewing muscles at the angle of the jaw (LMM & RMM). There are four bursts of energy expressed in microvolts.

The two on the left side are low intensity compared to the two bursts on the right. These exhibit relatively high intensity and greater symmetry and balance.

You don't need to be a doctor to see that there is a difference between the two traces in the image. The left two show very poor function, while the ones on the right show a much stronger, robust burst pattern. You want to have a result like the one on the right, not the left.

Transcutaneous Electric Nerve Stimulation

More specifically, this diagnostic tool is an Ultra-low Frequency Transcutaneous Electric Nerve Stimulator (ULFTNS). At a low rate of one pulse every 1.5 seconds or 40 per minute, your muscles are gently exercised. This is as opposed to the type of units seen on television infomercials which are high frequency devices that are intended to simply block the pain.

This device is intended to massage the muscles that are rich with nerves or that are fed by the Trigeminal nerve (Cranial Nerve V). The Trigeminal nerve is the largest and most complex of the cranial nerves in your head, and it takes part in processing the signals that go through the limbic system of your brain. That's what sets off your flight or fight response and is involved in stored and new emotional behavioral activity.

This kind of muscle stimulation acts as a massage that pumps out the stagnant lymphatic fluid and sluggish blood from the vessels in your muscle and energizes the cells at the same time. It's a similar concept as putting a trickle charge on a battery to get it back up to full strength.

Electrosonography

This method is also referred to simply as sonography because it uses vibration sensitive transducer technology that quickly and noninvasively records sounds and vibrations in your jaw joints.

To take this test, you wear lightweight sensors over your jaw joints. Then you open and close your mouth for a few cycles to record the sound. The computer software analyzes it to assess the condition of the internal workings of your jaw joints based on the sounds (vibrational signature). That lets us know much about the nature of a dysfunction if present.

I can also use electrosonography to monitor how effective your treatment program is. Then we can adjust your treatment accordingly.

Computerized Mandibular Scan

This diagnostic tool records "tracings" of the movement of your lower jaw (mandible) as it moves in time and space. The movement is captured by a sensor array that is worn on your head like a pair of glasses. The sensors contain eight small magnetometers.

For this test, a small magnet is applied to the teeth of your lower jaw just at your gum line. Various instructions are given to you about how to move your jaw so the motion can be recorded.

I can also use the mandibular scan along with the ULFTNS, mentioned above, to visualize the small, barely visible movements that take place while under involuntary control of the nerve stimulation pulse of the unit.

T-Scan

To measure tooth contact sequence and relative force generated during a bite, I use Tekscan's T-Scan®.

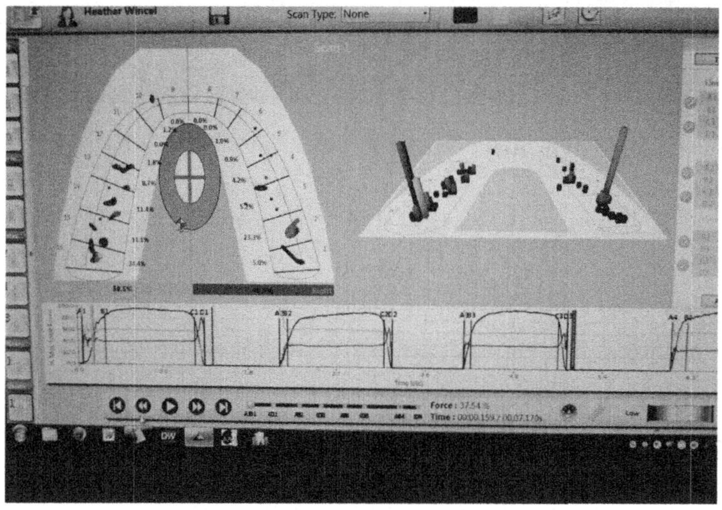

Demonstrating unequal forces before adjustment

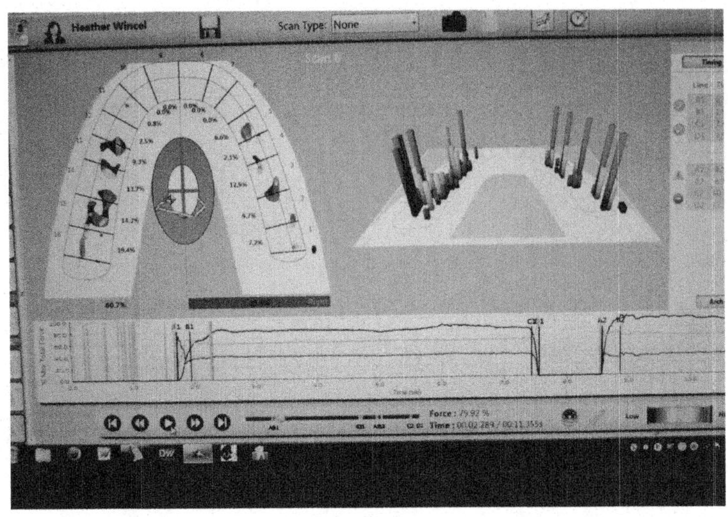

Demonstrating much greater balance of forces afterward

This is a marvelous device that can ferret out imbalances or high spots on your teeth. It's on a whole other level than the articulating paper that your dentist uses because the scan shows your bite in real-time action. You simply bite together and clench your teeth or move your jaw from side to side. Colorful bars dance on the computer screen as the timing, sequence and relative force of the contacts are displayed on the monitor. This tells me a lot about where and how hard your teeth are coming together when your jaw closes.

On the previous page are T-Scan graphs of the same patient. The first example is pre-adjustment, demonstrating unequal forces before the adjustment, and the companion image is the post-adjustment of the bite which shows much greater balance of forces and overall symmetry.

3D Radiography

Cone Beam Computed Tomography (CBCT) is not only helpful in diagnosing airway issues and cavitations, the use of the 3D scan can enable me to peer quite well into the inside of other bone structures of your head, neck and jaws.

Most dental scans are static units, meaning we do not capture data from a person who may be moving. In fact, movement can rarely be seen in an image.

But with 3D radiography, computerized mandibular scan, Acoustic Rhinometry, etc., I can understand what is happening and see how the movement of your jaw is affecting the interrelated systems in your face and neck.

Conclusion

Holistic dentists use these varied tests along with the thoughtful application of the treatment recommendations to help detoxify your body by making sure you are metal-free and free from infection while establishing a three-dimensional jaw postural relationship that balances your autonomic nervous system. These tests are important to discovering the status of your health and whether any of your systems are out of balance and need to be addressed.

I have found that some people are fascinated, motivated and ready to act while others are in denial that there is a problem in spite of ample evidence that something is going wrong. We become used to our own dysfunctions, and it's sometimes hard to imagine that what feels natural may not be best for you, and in fact, it could be setting off a series of other problems in your body.

All of us are in some state of accommodation or compensation to get through our life, but in my opinion, it's best to understand what's happening in our body so we can adjust our own situation accordingly. Once you do that, you may be able to tell how you've been affected not only physically but emotionally. Then you will see that you are not crazy for feeling the way you do, but your body is indeed driving you nuts.

End Notes

[1] "International College of Applied Kinesiology-USA." *ICAK-USA* |. Web. 29 Feb. 2016.

[2] Voll, Reinhard. *The measuring points of EAV on hands and feet.*ML-Verlag Uelzen (1989).

[3] "About Paracelsus, A Holistic Healthcare Center." *About Paracelsus, A Holistic Healthcare Center*. Web. 29 Feb. 2016.

[4] Bellack, Ervin., and P. J. Schouboe. "Rapid Photometric Determination of Fluoride in Water. Use of Sodium 2-(P -Sulfophenylazo)-1,8-dihydroxynaphthalene-3,6-disulfonate-Zirconium Lake." *Analytical Chemistry Anal. Chem.* 30.12 (1958): 2032-034.

[5] Lj, Kesić. "Normal Oral Flora - A New Classification - Part I." *Acta Stomatologica Naissi* 19.41 (March 2003).

CHAPTER 8

HEALTH-SUPPORTIVE MATERIALS AND PROCEDURES IN HOLISTIC DENTISTRY

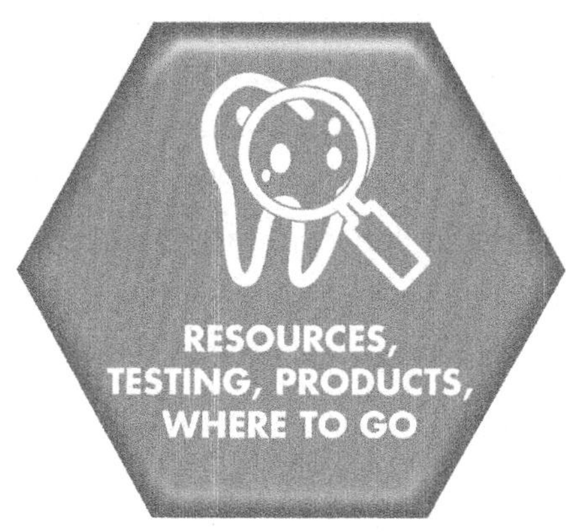

Now that you know that problems with your teeth, jaws and closely related structures may be causing a lot more problems than you realized, what do you do? Moving forward, you certainly don't want to jump out of the frying pan and into the fire. So first, you need to find and interview a doctor who you think can help you.

To find a holistic dentist, you can check with groups like the International Academy of Biological Dentistry and Medicine or do an Internet search for your area. Holistic dentists appreciate how your oral health and condition impacts your entire body, not just your teeth. They typically will promote their philosophy on their website. However, you have to be cautious because there aren't many holistic dentists around and you may find yourself having to travel to get the care you want and need.

Once you have identified a dentist who you think is qualified, then I suggest you take an active approach by interviewing them, asking multilevel questions to help you see if this is the person that you want to treat you. You can ask them about their techniques, philosophy and how they discover the underlying injury and conditions that are causing your problems. If your dentist understands the concept of the connection between your teeth and the ailments in the rest of your body, then they will be open to treating you as a whole person, not just a set of obvious dental issues.

Once you have selected a dentist, you will then have an in depth interview different from your initial interview of the doctor; a physical dental examination to assess your needs including the use of intra-oral photographs of your teeth, low dose radiation digital x-rays and even a Dental Materials Compatibility test. This gives the basic information necessary to begin to assemble a road map for your dental rejuvenation. For some it's a rejuvenation, while for others it can be a resurrection. Then in consultation with your doctor, you can establish a plan and suggested sequence of treatment, and together you can begin the process to resolve your issues.

You can also find reliable resources such as DrMercola.com which contains a wealth of information on almost all aspects of holistic health. Dr. Mercola is a voracious reader of research who is always on the lookout for valuable information to share with us. He does include a section on dentistry on his website, but it is not as global in scope as the contents of this book. Also you can consult my website www.DrNicholasMeyer.com for more information.

The following is a list of health supportive materials and procedures that are mentioned in this book that are arranged in alphabetical order for easy reference.

Cavitations

The traditional way of dealing with a cavitation, a diseased area of your jaw bone, is through surgical treatment (see Chapter 5 – Root Canals & Jaw Bone Lesions: Hidden Causes of Disease). I, like other holistic dentists, rely on surgery to remove the necrotic areas of a cavitation to allow for your bone to heal and regenerate. This entails scraping the abscesses and infected tissue from the healthy bone.

It is extremely important that the surgical site is irrigated with various solutions to aid in the removal of bacteria and toxins. Then to assist with bone regeneration, platelet-rich fibrin (PRF) alone or along with a reabsorbable membrane to guide new bone growth can be placed in the surgical wound site. The area is closed with sutures that help prevent bacterial growth.

Another valuable adjunctive tool used at this time is a high-energy laser (Nd:YAG). This high-energy laser can denature the pathologic proteins (diseased tissues) and bacteria in the lesion, and help cause a stable thermal activated blood clot to form.

Another one of my preferred treatments to encourage the bone to regenerate is low-level laser therapy (LLLT). Here the laser therapy has a bio-stimulation effect that re-energizes the cells and their microstructures, including the mitochondria that live inside your cells, giving you an enhanced ability to heal. You can also have less pain and swelling.

The benefit of the low-level laser therapy is that as it re-energizes your tissues, Nitric Oxide (NO) is produced. Nitric Oxide relaxes smooth muscle tissue, dilates your lymphatic tissue, increases collagen production, reduces swelling and is an anti-bacterial agent. Nitric Oxide is a very small and very important, body-friendly molecule composed of single atoms of nitrogen and oxygen that acts as a signalling molecule in your system to stimulate other important chemical reactions to take place in the cell.

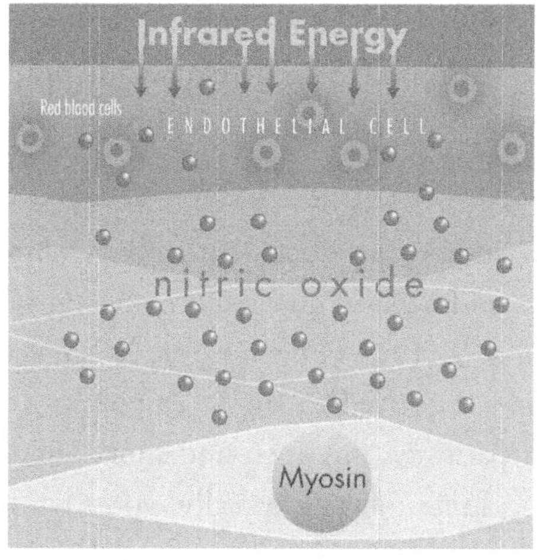

Laser Therapy sends infrared energy into your tissues

Another therapy I use on cavitations is ozone therapy. Prolozone™ treatment involves injections of collagen-producing substances and ozone gas into the damaged connective tissue in and around your joints. It lessens the pain as it helps your ligaments repair themselves.

Another way that can help control bacterial infections is through Hyperbaric Oxygen Therapy (HBOT). HBOT is used to increase the oxygen tension inside your damaged oxygen-depleted tissue. By providing more oxygen, it kills the bacteria that can't live on oxygen. It also improves the circulation in the area and allows new bone and vascular tissue to grow and fill in the space.

I also suggest homeopathic therapy to support the tissues not only with cavitation surgery but with other surgeries in your mouth. Homeopathic therapies can assist in your lymphatic drainage, support your liver for detoxification purposes, give you an overall general body healing and well-being, and support new bone growth and soft tissue healing.

There are several products, including enzymes, natural antimicrobials and healing nutrients that can give you systemic support prior to and after the surgery. In some cases, limited antibiotics may be needed. It is important that all body detoxification pathways are open and functioning well: bowels, kidneys, skin, lungs, and especially your lymphatic system. Electrolyte balance is also important for detoxification, healing, and ease in administering IV sedation.

Intravenous Vitamin C (IV-C) can also assist with healing by helping to clean up the toxic materials and bacteria released into your bloodstream during treatment.

Dental Devices

Typically dental devices are created to treat orthodontics, missing teeth, TMD problems and airway issues (see Chapter 4 – TMD and Airway Disorders: I Haven't Got Time for the Pain). The design of a dental appliance is limited only by the imagination of the doctor and the needs of your mouth and teeth. There are a myriad of ways in which the various materials can be put together to achieve the goal we have set for your mouth.

As an example, I created a long term removable orthosis for a patient that was somewhat jokingly nicknamed the Starship

Enterprise, owing to its unique design and choice of materials. An orthosis is a device that provides for biomechanical alignment. It was a work of art, never to be duplicated again because it fulfilled the unique needs of this man. He has worn it successfully for well over 10 years at the time of this writing and it fully resolved his bite issues.

Another example is a device created to change a child's alveolar process by encouraging the arch of the roof of their mouth to expand so there is enough room for teeth to erupt.

Still other dental devices are designed to reposture the mandible (lower jaw) into a different position to relieve excessive pressure within the temporomandibular joint when dealing with TMD. Other devices are designed to reposition your tongue so that it has greater room in the back of your throat to treat snoring or obstructive sleep apnea.

One of the dental devices I recommend is the FDA-approved Nociceptive Trigeminal Inhibition-Tension Suppression System (NTI-TSS). This is a rather unique little device that is successfully used to prevent the development of migraine headaches. It turns out that most migraine headaches are caused by excess muscle contraction by your temporalis muscles. By turning off the muscle before it can overwork, you can turn off the reason why migraines start.

Another useful dental device is a nighttime bite guard. This device is designed to only be worn at night to interrupt your teeth from grinding and inflicting damaging forces against one another and the muscles of your face. Nighttime bite guards are made for either the upper jaw or the lower jaw, but I prefer to treat the lower jaw.

These devices can be purchased in pharmacies or custom crafted for your mouth. The custom-made devices are less bulky and therefore you're more apt to wear them compared to an over-the-counter type. But the store-bought device costs a fraction of what a custom-made one does. So if you can wear the store-bought device and it protects your teeth from grinding, then I'm all for it. If neither is worn however, the damage from grinding teeth can be severe and the costs very high to restore your health.

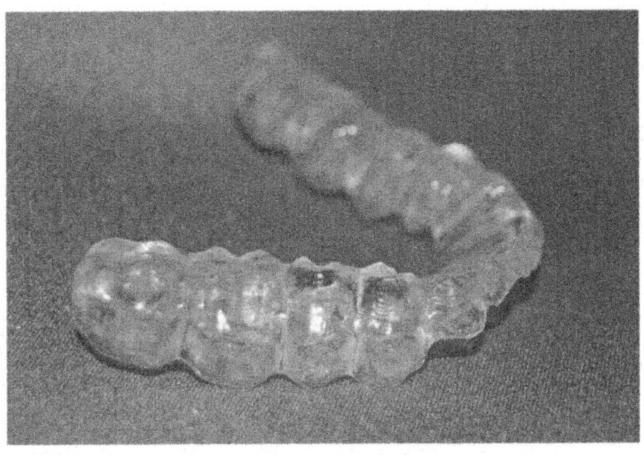

Lower jaw nighttime bite guard

Fluoride

There are a wide range of issues that contribute to the formation of caries (cavities) in the teeth, including the pH balance of your mouth and the food that you eat. There aren't any one or two dental products that alone will prevent tooth decay. However, there are many products that will go a long way to help prevent tooth decay by controlling the environment in your mouth.

The most important thing to remember is to use toothpaste without fluoride (see Chapter 3 – Fluoride: More Foe than Friend?). In order to do that, you have to read the labels on toothpaste tubes. Virtually all of the major name brands contain fluoride as the active ingredient. There is one of the more popular healthy brands that's often thought to be free of fluoride, but to be sure, read the label.

Also be sure to request that your dentist use dental materials without fluoride. That includes the mouth rinse. If you have a holistic dentist who is following the results of your compatibility test, then you shouldn't have to worry about this issue.

If you're considering a fluoride-removing home water system, many home water treatment systems are ineffective with many of the more harmful substances, including fluoride. Their common claims are for removing certain parasitic organisms such as Cryptococcus and Cryptosporidium, among others; they remove harmful lead and chlorine that can create certain by-products that are linked to cancer and they also remove sediment, odor, pesticides, dioxins, chloroform and petrochemicals.

Basic reverse osmosis (RO) systems used to treat water can cause the water to become non-vital (lacking electrons & mineral deficient). The water produced is shifted to the acid side of the pH scale (<7), while in nature, running water gives up electrons readily and is on the alkaline side of the pH scale. Keep in mind that the pH scale is logarithmic. This means that each number is altered by a factor of 10. This is a big deal, and unless you know this, you can be fooled by the absolute number on the scale.

The more desirable water treatment units have the following characteristics: they remove fluoride; create micro-clusters of water; the water is produced in an alkaline state; has a high oxidative reduction potential (ORP) value (the ability to carry a charge); and has minerals within it that allows a charge to pass through it. The top end units can also remove the volatile organic compounds (VOC).

And one more note about alkaline water. Please do not drink water, in general and alkaline water especially, during your meal time. Do not drink it at least 15 minutes prior and at least an hour afterward. The alkalinity of the water will neutralize the stomach acid that is necessary to activate the enzymes that digest your foods, especially the more difficult to break down proteins in your meal. Additionally hormonal signaling in the stomach becomes faulty and a whole cascade of other metabolic challenges comes into play.

One purpose of the water is to flush your body's systems and to help load you up on a source rich in electrons. However, your primary source of electrons should be your whole foods, and walking out on the soil and in the sun, without overdoing it.

Mercury Removal

After finding a qualified holistic dentist, you can safely remove mercury-containing materials from your teeth such as metal fillings (see Chapter 2 – Heavy Metal… And Not the Rock Band Kind!). Ideally the doctor will give you a Dental Materials Compatibility test and review with you the selection of dental materials that will be used, as per the results of your compatibility test.

In my practice, I tend to honor your body's natural immune cycle of 7-14-21 days. Simply put, we do not want to perform mercury amalgam removal on the same day of the week on successive weeks. Instead I prefer to stagger the days to avoid the cycle. If not, you can cause harm by unnecessarily challenging your body.

Here's how I remove the mercury from your teeth. First I use a non-vasoactive dental anesthetic to numb the tissue. Next I administer a homeopathic mercury detox rinse. This is a type of homeopathic remedy that can bind up (chelate) loose mercury with other molecules that are then carried out of your body either through urine or feces. These remedies come in liquid, spray or pellet form.

Next I apply a rubber dam to the teeth in question. This provides a good barrier, though not a perfect one, to contain the debris that is generated during the removal of the filling.

You are then fitted with a nasal hood that allows oxygen to flow under positive pressure. Finally, the dam fabric is coated with a thick hand cream that also has a mercury chelator which grabs any metal ions it encounters. This will help to bind the debris that comes loose in the removal process.

There are also preparations that are taken outside of your mouth. Both the doctor and assistant don protective special mercury vapor masks to save them from breathing the vapor that is liberated during the extraction. Next an extra-oral High Efficiency Particulate Arresting (HEPA) vacuum is placed near the operating field and turned on. And finally, a negative ion generator is turned on so that your immediate environment is kept as scrubbed as possible from errant mercury.

Once all of these preparations are in place, the procedure commences. The filling is removed as much as possible in large segments to limit the amount of small particles or breakdown debris of the material. Any decay or cavities that have formed around the filling are also removed.

Then the tooth is cleaned of residual oxide of mercury that is left at the new edges. This leftover material, if not completely removed, hinders the new bond of the restorative filling material to the tooth.

Once the tooth is deemed as clean, depending on the amount of teeth involved, I will complete the restorations with the dam still in place. There really isn't a right or wrong way. In my practice, I am fairly divided between either technique, and I allow prevailing circumstances to direct the flow of the appointment. Regardless, once the dam is removed, you are thoroughly rinsed out and given an additional oral chelation rinse that is the same as the first one you take prior to the placement of the rubber dam.

At that point, your teeth are then treated with ozone to thoroughly disinfect and desensitize the exposed tooth surface. The new restoration is then placed with substances that are compatible with your body chemistry as per your Dental Materials Compatibility test. This includes direct and indirect restoration of your teeth with mercury-free materials that are chosen from the list of safe materials and then used according to the manufacturers' recommendations.

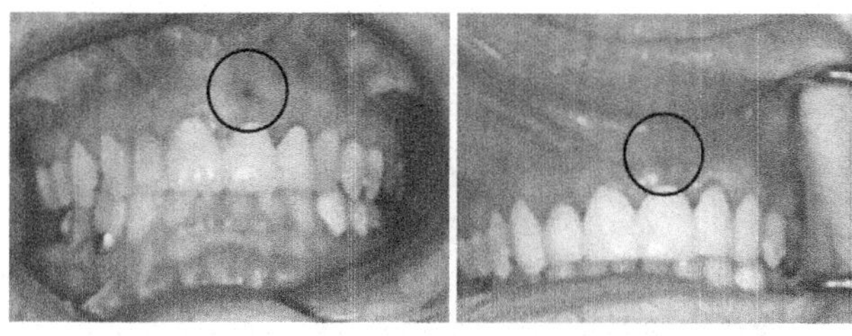

Mercury pigment tattooing on left and restored on the right

The Dental Materials Compatibility test gives you results for literally thousands of materials for all kinds of dental use. So if you need an impression taken of your tooth for a dental cap rather than a filling, materials will be chosen from this list.

I also consider these materials in terms of longevity. You want to have a material that has a reasonably long life. I have seen mercury fillings in patients' mouths that are over 50 years old. Yes, that's right: 50+ years old. I'm not advocating this kind of long-term exposure to mercury but this material does last for long periods of time. Dental gold also has a history of longevity for both single tooth replacement as well as multiple teeth replacements, as in a fixed bridge or the framework for a removable partial denture. Again we strive to be non-metallic and immune system friendly.

Many people ask about on-going detox practices. I encourage everyone to take something. Those in my area I will encourage to see other health care providers to assess and monitor their heavy metal detoxification. Not everyone follows along with that. The following image illustrates several (not all) of currently available over the counter preparations for heavy metal removal.

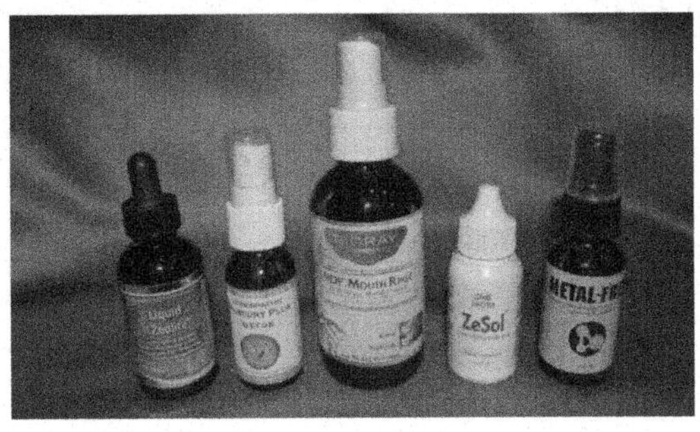

A sampling of detoxification products

Periodontal Disease

Traditional dentists typically rely on root planing (scraping of the teeth) and then later, open flap surgery to treat periodontal disease. However, I believe the correct holistic dentistry solution is laser assisted gum treatment (see Chapter 6 – Periodontal Disease: Beware the Biofilm). Laser treatment is kinder to your body because it is much less invasive and therefore less painful than the more traditional method of surgery. Pain is readily managed with homeopathic remedies or mild analgesics.

I use a laser that removes debris from your gum, including diseased tissue and pathologic proteins. I can actually feel the roughness on your tooth through the fiber optic cable.

Next I use a combination of ultrasonic scalers with irrigants and hand instruments to cleanse the root surface of the accumulated layers. Once the tooth is deemed to be clean, the laser is used to sterilize the pocket and cause a coagulum (clot) to form. Recent research (2015) has confirmed that the use of a particular wavelength laser (1064µm) can kill almost all pathogens (harmful bacteria) in the gum pocket.

Then I use my finger to compress the gum tissues against the tooth. A stable fibrin clot forms at the gingival crest of your gum. Once this coagulum heals, it becomes the new attachment between the bone and the tooth.

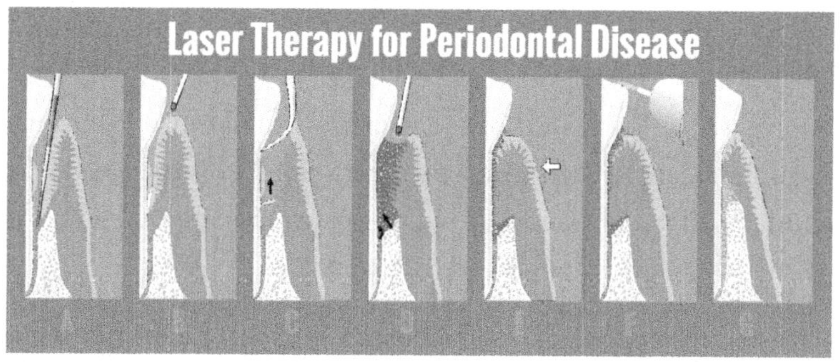

The area is cleaned, scraped, lasered to form a clot then compressed

Then, if necessary (usually), your tooth is filed down using a high-speed hand drill and diamond burr, to prevent occlusal trauma, which is pressure from too high a tooth.

Another treatment I've found to be beneficial on advanced periodontal disease is ozone infusion of the gum. Ozone is O_3, a potent gas that is antimicrobial, anti-fungal and anti-viral. By infusing pure ozone gas around your teeth and gums, I can treat the deepest of periodontal pockets. The ozone is delivered through specialized dental trays that have been custom made to conform to your mouth and teeth. There is an "in" port and "out" port that creates the free exchange of the gas. See photo below.

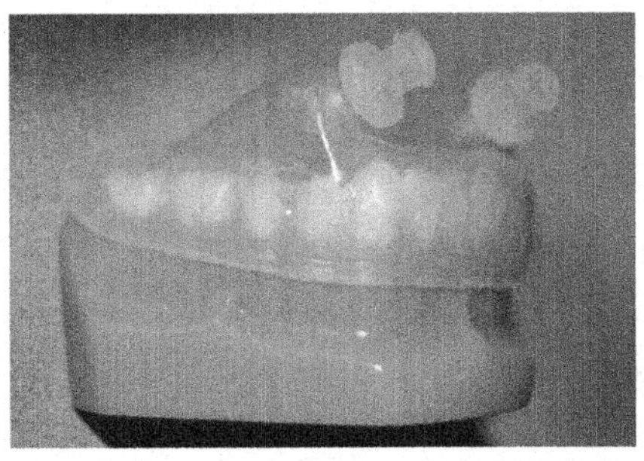

An ozone dental tray

Along with laser and ozone therapy, sometimes additional treatments are needed to manage periodontal disease, including gum grafting and bone grafting using artificial, animal donor or tissue taken from elsewhere in your body.

I may also utilize platelet-rich plasma (PRP) that is from your own blood plasma that has been manipulated in a centrifuge to cause it to be enriched with your own platelets. PRP contain growth factors and stem cells that stimulate the healing of your tissues. Fortunately, this isn't needed often for the procedure I just described. This procedure can enhance a number of different dental therapies, not just periodontal disease.

Another beneficial treatment for periodontal disease is called oil pulling. This therapy (remedy) has its origins in the Ayurveda health system in India hundreds of years ago. In this treatment, you vigorously froth organic sesame oil or coconut oil in your mouth by forcefully swishing it around your teeth. The action of the oil causes a disruption of the cell membrane and the death of microbes. The oil must be swished vigorously for about 15 minutes to be really effective and improve the tone of your tissue. It is best performed in the morning.

I suggest a simple system: take 1 teaspoon of organic sesame oil or coconut, place it into your mouth and begin the swishing. It's a good idea to combine this with a morning shower and use the time constructively for both activities. If you time it well, you can finish your shower at the same time you need to spit out the oil. The soap from your shower will emulsify the oil and help disperse it and you can use the shower water to rinse your mouth after the swishing.

A large number of my patients use this technique and I am usually quite amazed at how toned their tissue looks and how clean their teeth appear. However in the most advanced cases of periodontitis, unfortunately the oil may not get down deep enough into the "pocket" or the defect between the tooth and gum to be as beneficial.

Lastly, the use of a probiotic tooth paste can be beneficial for those sufferers of periodontal disease. Probiotics are live microorganisms, usually bacteria, that are similar to beneficial microorganisms found in the human gut.

Other Healthy Materials and Procedures

I also like to use craniosacral therapy, which is a wonderful treatment therapy that is an offshoot of chiropractic techniques. This therapy is designed to unwind the soft tissue of your body that is holding your bones in the wrong place, causing subsequent skeletal accommodations. This is one of my personal favorite therapies either by itself or coupled with treatment for TMD. In fact, I have had people who are able to terminate their active TMD therapy after several sessions with a skilled craniosacral therapist.

CHAPTER 9

HEALTHY EATING, HEALTHY TEETH

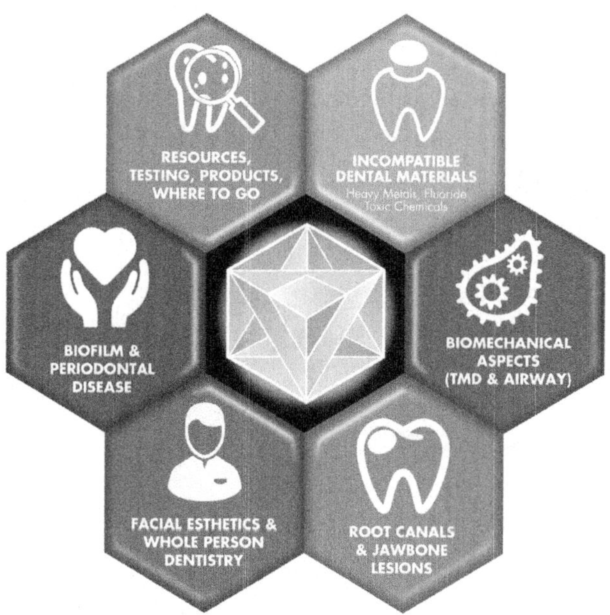

This chapter is for all readers… whether you feel you or your loved ones have minor concerns or any of the more complex problems shown on my Holistic Dental Matrix™.

When we look at tooth decay, it's actually an infection of the tooth. A tooth is the hardest structure in the human body and yet this kind of infection can turn it into mush. Part of how susceptible you are to this process depends on how well your tooth protein matrix developed and was calcified.

We all know that tooth decay comes with inadequate brushing and flossing. That's because brushing and flossing physically remove the bacteria from your teeth that is known as plaque. So in other words, we control the external environment to prevent tooth decay.

However, there are other factors that contribute to tooth decay (caries). One viewpoint was developed in the 1960s by Dr. Ralph Steinman of Loma Linda School of Dentistry who meticulously studied the flow of fluid in teeth.[1]

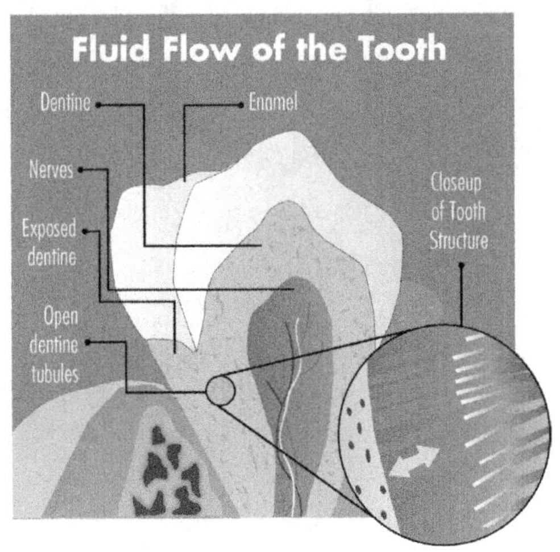

Microtubules can carry bacteria into the surrounding bone

Dr. Steinman determined that a healthy tooth is a closed high pressure system. He found through experiments that the "lymph" from the pulp chamber of the tooth migrated, under pressure, to the outside of the tooth where it is attached to the ligament in your mouth which holds it in place.

As long as there is a positive fluid pressure from the inside to the outside, bacteria cannot enter and live in the microscopic tubules of the tooth. However, Dr. Steinman discovered that once sugar was eaten by the subject, this pump actually reversed and acted like suction so that the bacteria could now enter into the tooth. Further, he found that this control mechanism was under the control of a "parotid hormone." This hormone was found to be the gate keeper for the direction of the fluid flow within the tooth.

This direct connection between problems in your teeth and what you eat can be seen in the Meridian tooth chart, which is based on traditional Chinese medicine beliefs about the way your life-force flows through your body. Looking at the energetic relationship of each tooth, you can see which teeth relate to each part of your body.

For example, a mid-teen came to me for an examination. He had exemplary dental health with virtually not a scrap of plaque to be found. However, a cavity was identified. Upon treatment of this cavity, it opened up into a large lesion that almost defied explanation as to what caused it.

The teenager was sent for energetic analysis and a high amount of inflammation was found within his intestines. This corresponded to the acupuncture meridian that connected to the tooth in question. It turned out that the teenager was indulging in foods that were highly inflammatory to his gut and thus the tooth. In this case, his cavity turned out to be a bellwether of a deeper problem that would have gone on for quite a while before surfacing into a much more serious type of illness.

That's why our health is said to begin in our gut. The whole field of Naturopathic Medicine is based on that basic tenant. When your gut is not right, you are not right. With respect to your teeth and your gut, the most important thing to remember is to shun sugar in almost all forms lest you turn the parotid hormone pump on inside your body and cause the fluid flow of your teeth to reverse direction and cause tooth decay.

Healthy Eating

This book isn't meant to be a comprehensive guide to foods. Book shelves are full of books that are dedicated to this topic. I'd like to provide only the more basic guidelines for healthy eating for healthy teeth.

The first rule of healthy eating is to eat as close to nature as you can. Your food selections need to ideally include a wide variety of vegetables, both above the ground type and those that grow underground.

Furthermore, they need to be from the whole palette of colors available from nature. We humans begin eating with our eyes and our noses. This sets the internal stage to prepare our body for the digestive process that follows. Your mouth and teeth are the physical start of your digestion.

When we eat, the most important thing we are feeding is our brain. This is brought home when you realize that although our brain is only between 2-3 percent of our body weight, it consumes approximately 25 percent of our energy. Another consideration about our brain is that, according to modern research, more of our brain resides in our gut than in the space between our ears. So, you can perhaps appreciate that we are directly feeding our gut-brain directly when we eat.

For further discussions on the merits of one type of diet over another type of diet, I suggest you do some minimal research to begin the inquiry process within that arena. It is far too complex an area to barely touch upon in this book.

Eat P.A.C.O.

According to what I have learned in multiple research studies, the principles I use to help guide healthy eating is P.A.C.O.:

Primitive

Alkaline

Colorful

Organic

These principles will help you to prevent cancer, heart disease, diabetes and many other illnesses. They will help you maintain a healthy weight and feel vibrant and alive into your golden years.

Eating "primitive" means eating less processed foods like packaged meals and snack food like chips and sweets. It means eating more food that comes straight from the farm to the table. Take milk, for example. Pasteurization removes the healthy parts of milk products in order to make it safe for transportation and storage. Plenty of people drink milk thinking that it's healthy for them, yet humans are the only species to consume milk from another species after they are weaned from their mother's breast. Raw milk and raw cheeses are much better for you that their processed counterparts.

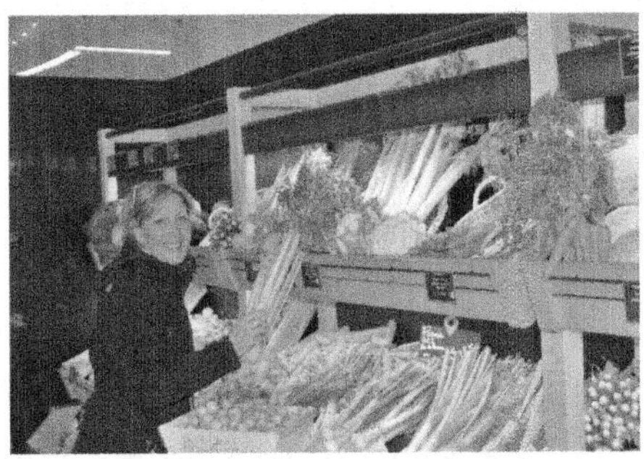

Nancy eating P.A.C.O.

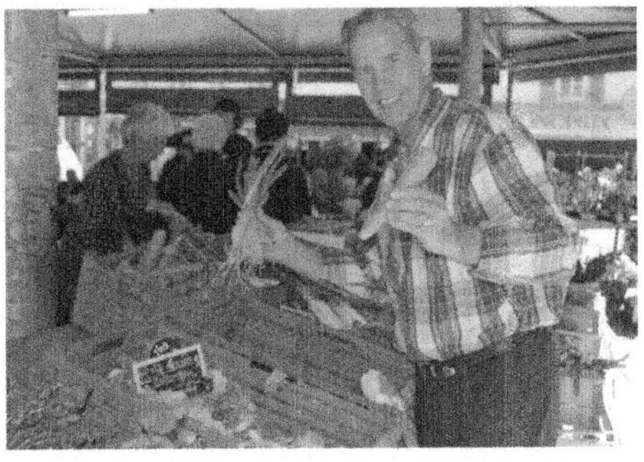

I eat P.A.C.O., too

Eating "alkaline" means keeping a good ratio between acidic foods, which are animal-based foods, and alkaline or plant-based food. Humans are designed to be alkaline with an intracellular pH at about 7.35-7.45. Shifting to alkaline foods decreases inflammation in your blood and tissues.

Tooth decay or cavities occur in an acidic environment, so one set of foods that helps balance the pH levels in your mouth are certain cheeses like aged cheddar, Swiss, mozzarella and Monterey Jack. When eaten alone as a snack or at the end of a meal, these cheeses stimulate saliva flow, which clears the mouth of food debris and neutralizes harmful acids.

Eating "colorful" means that you need to focus on food that is naturally green, red, yellow, orange and purple for at least 6-7 servings a day. This will provide important minerals and vitamins for your body in a natural way, along with fiber which is essential for good gut health. Orange-colored vegetables, such as sweet potatoes, pumpkin, carrots and winter squash in particular are loaded with beta-carotene (Vitamin A), an essential nutrient for healthy teeth and gum tissue.

To me, eating "organic" means avoiding foods that are farmed with pesticides and do not contain genetically modified organisms (GMO). Virtually all commercial GMOs are engineered to withstand the direct application of herbicide and/or to produce an insecticide themselves. Since this is engineered into the food, you're consuming these molecules along with the food. Research has shown that the body does not know how to process these substances that look like foods you know but are not the food of your ancestors.

The current trend toward hybridizing and genetic modification is one of the reasons for the huge increase in gluten intolerance seen in many people. And it's not just grains that are affected. Did you know that many of the products in grocery stores contain genetically modified organisms? Many aren't even labeled for GMOs nor are they required to be labeled.

One easy way to change your eating habits right now is try to do most of your shopping on the perimeter of the store instead of the aisles. Usually the processed foods are in the center in the boxes, cans and freezer section of your super market.

Calcium

The one supplement you hear about most when it comes to your teeth is calcium. We know that taking calcium supplements can help your teeth and bones. But is that really true? In fact, calcium supplements can't replace the lack of calcium in your diet because it turns out that it's the wrong form of calcium.

Dr. Thomas Levy, in *Death by Calcium*, asserts that we, as a nation, are already given too much calcium in our food and that we have a great deal of illness as a result.[2] Drinking milk, as it is commonly available today, also does not give us the same nutrients as it once did prior to pasteurization. The exception being raw milk.

Pasteurization is intended to destroy certain disease-carrying germs and prevent milk from souring. This is done by keeping the milk at a temperature of 145 degrees to 150 degrees F for half an hour, and then reducing the temperature to not more than 55 degrees F. This unfortunately destroys useful bacteria and nutritional constituents as well. The worst thing pasteurization does is make insoluble the major part of the calcium contained in raw milk.

The best way to get the calcium your teeth need is to eat lots of green vegetables like collard greens, broccoli, kale, edamame, bok choy and okra. Proteins such as sardines, salmon, tofu, white beans and almonds are also good sources of calcium, along with figs and oranges, which have an added benefit because of their vitamin C content which helps prevent gingivitis.

Digestion

Our physical digestion begins in the mouth, so what we put in our mouth and the health of our mouth affects how our food is digested. You also have to keep in mind that a healthy immune system relies on a healthy gut—that's where more than 70 percent of our immune function develops. And your mouth is the beginning of your gut.

The enzymes in our saliva begin the process of digestion by breaking down starch and moistening the food. Your teeth chew to break down the food so there's more of a surface area for digestive enzymes in your stomach and intestines. When your teeth are damaged or your bite is challenged, that has an effect on how well you can digest food because it isn't being adequately broken down. When you lose teeth and shifting takes place, the remaining teeth just aren't as efficient.

Can we live without teeth? Yes, of course. But that comes at a steep price. You get fewer nutrients readily available for your gut to absorb because you cannot chew your food properly and efficiently. Supplemental digestive enzymes are important for most people to take to aid in the digestion of our foods.

Your mouth also signals your nervous and hormonal systems when you eat. This instructs the liver to produce bile and your stomach to produce acid. One way to optimize your digestion is to minimize or not even drink liquids while eating because it dilutes your stomach acids. If you adequately chew your food to mix with your own saliva the mass turns into a somewhat slushy paste that is easily swallowed and more able to be digested at the next step. We need the stomach acids to help kill the bacteria we consumed in our food, and the acids further break down the slushy food so it can be processed and absorbed through our small intestine.

Drinking while eating can interfere with the natural and necessary levels of bile and stomach acid. The bile by the way is what is used to emulsify the fats in our diet. It is appropriate here to say that eating fats don't make you fat. That is a whole different subject best left to books on that subject. But I will say that you need to eat fats to survive in an optimally healthy way. Low fat diets can actually contribute to illness.

So, if you drink while you eat, your digestion process slows down, allowing for the build-up of toxic waste even if you're eating healthy foods. However, drinking water (non-alkaline) more than 30 minutes before and after you eat can help your digestion.

Leaky gut syndrome, a condition where your intestines are more permeable, means that the cells that line the intestinal wall aren't joined well together. This allows larger undigested molecules along with toxic substances to leak into your blood stream. This in turn prompts your white blood cells to multiply to fight the "infection" in your blood, which in turn ramps up your system to the point where it becomes exhausted and is not able to fight other types of infections. It puts your entire body into a perpetual fight or flight mode, which stresses all of your vital organs. So from a dental perspective, this can be avoided by having sound teeth, a balance of forces in the mouth, foods that are well chewed and mixed well with saliva for optimal utilization by the body.

The way your digestive system absorbs food is fairly well-understood. You can see an extensive diagram below that outlines the absorption of the various foods.

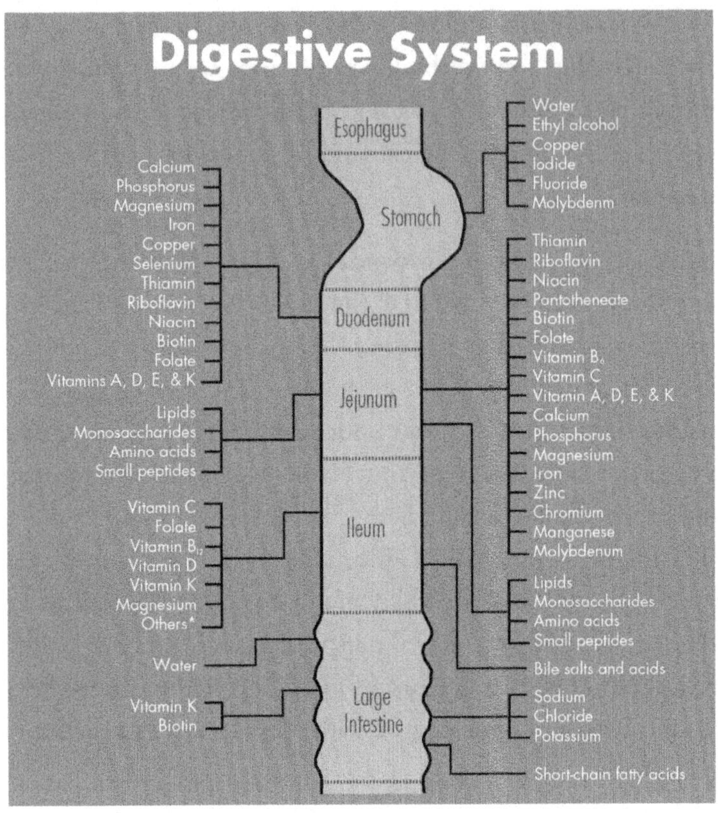

Where essential vitamins and minerals are absorbed

However, for some people, one of the main culprits of gut inflammation is gluten. Gluten can cause your gut cells to release zonulin, a protein that can break apart the tight junctions in your intestinal lining. For other people, infections, stress, age and a build-up of toxins can also cause these tight junctions to break apart. Restore® is a product that has the ability to heal your gut by tightening your gut junctions.

Toxins

There have been documented studies by the Environmental Working Group which have found over 300 chemicals and toxins in the average adult.[3] There are also more than 278 chemicals and toxins in the cord blood of newborn infants according to the EWG's benchmark investigation of industrial chemicals, pollutants and pesticides in umbilical cord blood: "Body Burden: Pollution in Newborns." Is it any wonder childhood cancer is on the rise?

Removing the toxins from your system is a good way to get your body back into balance. Your body becomes weaker when it encounters molecules that it wasn't designed to handle. These molecules include toxins you eat in your food, such as steroids, antibiotics, hormones and genetically modified organisms.

We are also exposed to toxins in our environment that are locked into our body. Things like lead, arsenic, mercury, ozone, aldehydes, carbon monoxide and particulate matter.

The process of removing toxins, such as lead or mercury, from your bloodstream is done by means of a chelate. A chelate is a chemical compound that contains a metal ion attached to at least two nonmetal ions. It's a natural process that removes the metal toxins from your system. Your cells can produce some of these substances but if there are too many of them or the innate mechanisms are not working well, extra help is needed.

Products like ACZ Nano Extra Strength®, a simple oral spray, has been shown to increase urinary output of mercury up to 103,500 percent over baseline during only 12 hours of post-provocation urine collection. This can also cause an array of challenging systemic symptoms so you are advised to seek the services of a skilled practitioner. Other forms of detoxification are by ingestion or IV infusions of various chelating substances, herbal foot patches, ionic foot baths, infra-red sauna, dry body scrub, among other methods.

Probiotics

You may not know it but we have a second brain in our guts that is created by the massive volume of bacteria that live there termed the human microbiome. This is a sophisticated and helpful bacterial congregation that communicates with our body and vice-versa through an estimated 500 million nerves and 20 different types of neurons that are in our gut. This conglomeration includes autonomous microcircuits, chemical and mechanical sensing, control of muscle movement as well as the secretion of hormones and enzymes.

Over two million unique bacterial genes are found in each human microbiome. Since the gut begins with the mouth, that's one of the reasons why the human bite is one of the worst wounds you can get, because of the diverse bacteria present in it.

Vast amounts of money have been recently devoted to researching the human microbiome. It is believed that because of the vastness of the microbial biome that our DNA is actually more bacterial in nature than "human." That's why some research suggests that we are a microbiome hosting a human form. It is estimated that there are between some 23,000 to 1 trillion sets of genes creating who we are. These findings may necessitate a redefining of what it is to be human. So far we've barely scratched the surface of this most important recognition by modern science, but these scientific findings support the work of Naturopathic Physicians who have always held that our health begins in the gut.

To sustain healthy gut bacteria, first we need to balance the pH of our system. When there is an imbalance in the pH, the microflora (biome) goes out of balance and can lead to an overgrowth of Candida. This is yeast that is responsible for disease such as bloating, anal itching and more.

Also within the gut there are multitudes of areas that have their own microclimate and thus their own pH requirements. This is how we can explain the huge diversity of bacteria in the gut, where everything about it is dependent on the pH of the local environment.

We see similar microclimates in the mouth and thus a wide diversity of bacteria. When bad bacteria take over, the result can be tooth decay or its cousin, gum disease.

Imbalances occur when we either do not adequately masticate our food, drink too much of a beverage when we dine, eat too much of the wrong foods like carbonated beverages sweetened with high fructose corn syrup or coffee. When this imbalance occurs, the body is robbed of vital nutrients like minerals. This is true for any area of the gut, but in the mouth you see this showing up in the form of some type of disease because of the complicated surface energies and interactions between the systems of your teeth.

One of the paths to well-being is to eat to restore and retain the balance of our intestinal bacteria. We need to include in our diet foods that aren't too clean. I know, I almost can't believe that I am saying this either, but we need to have some dirty foods. "Why?" you ask. It turns out that the dirt in our fruits and vegetables carry the very bacteria that we need for gut health and thus our own health.

There are new products available in the marketplace that can help to restore your disturbed biome. The ones I recommend are Restore and Megaspore Biotics.

End Notes

[1]Steinman, Ralph R. "Pharmacologic Control of Dentinal Fluid Movement and Dental Caries in Rats." *Journal of Dental Research* 47 (September 1968): 5720-724.

[2] Levy, Thomas E. *Death By Calcium.* Medfox Publishing 1st edition (2013).

[3] Environmental Working Group. "Body Burden: Pollution in Newborns." EWG (July 14, 2005).implants? A systematic review." *Clin Implant Dent Relat Res.* 15.1 (February, 2013): 47-52.

CHAPTER 10

FACIAL ESTHETICS: HOW TO GET YOUR LIGHTS TURNED ON

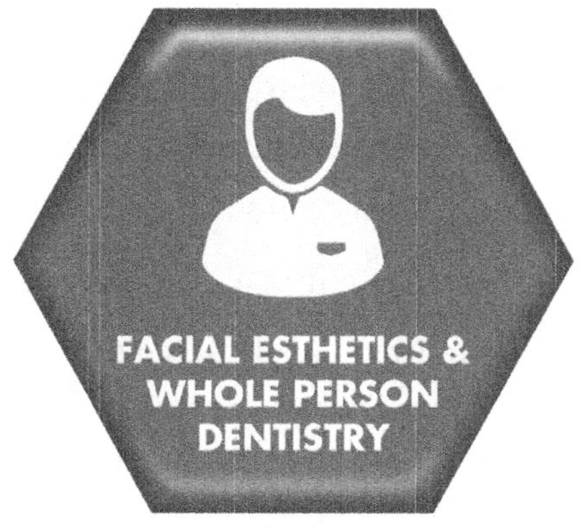

Ah, the search for perpetual youth, the siren-call of the aging. Our obsession with looking youthful and being our best has been around for centuries if not millennia. Everyone knows how Ponce de Leon searched Florida for the fabled "Fountain of Youth."

Today we are closer than ever to achieving that goal. The baby boom generation is seeing to that. The fountain of youth is not a place or in a single treatment, but is found in the components of healthy living and thoughtfully applied science.

This chapter is a brief introduction into the potpourri of what could best be termed Natural or Holistic Facial Esthetics. I have seen miracles in facial esthetics from reposturing (balancing) the head, neck and jaws through the techniques outlined in Chapter 4 – TMD & Airway. You see, when these structures are well balanced spatially, you benefit in many ways. The autonomic nervous system has to compensate less so it works better, allowing a greater flow of nervous information and circulation to all parts of your system. The people who undergo this therapy literally light up! Their eyes become enlivened, greater energy occurs naturally and there is a greater bounce in their step.

That said, there are also folks who do not need to have their jaw repostured. Their need involves their life support system, the skin and not the skeletal support system. Then too there are those who benefit from both or those who have some skeletal deficiency and still require attention to both elements.

The treatment involves minimally or noninvasive techniques such as various frequency devices that use light and sound as well as micro-current devices. These are healthy techniques whereas the Vampire Facelift®, Botox™ (natural but unhealthy), Restyln and others of that ilk just cannot get the job done if there is a postural imbalance that "short circuits" the autonomic nervous system. You can enhance the skin's tightness with them through either tightening the muscle or stimulating the production of collagen. Thus, you can enhance the glow and texture of the skin, but you cannot derive the same benefit that the jaw reposturing treatment can.

By the way, I was the first dentist to offer Vampire Facelifts in Scottsdale. This is done by drawing blood from the patient and spinning it in a centrifuge to separate out the platelets, which are then injected back under the patient's facial skin. It can also be combined with other fillers.

You achieve a much greater, more optimized appearance through a combination of both types of techniques. Furthermore, the foods and supplements and other "vices" we may enjoy, such as smoking and alcoholic consumption, will vastly influence the internal terrain of our skin. That's because our skin is our life support barrier system, and is also known as the third kidney. It is the largest excretory organ of the body. So really, it is crucial for optimal skin care that we humans have a regular detox regimen in place to help this complex organ from the inside out and keep it functioning.

My patients have had phenomenal life-changing outcomes through holistic facial esthetics. Their treatments were not specifically undertaken with the goal of rejuvenating their appearance but to enhance their jaw posture to relieve TMD pain or improve their airway due to snoring or sleep apnea.

But it is obvious, even to the most casual observer, that holistic dentistry changes lives and at so many levels and on many dimensions. The wear and tear of sun damage and city living require a different care and treatment.

K.W. Testimonial

I was referred to Dr. Meyer by my homeopathic physician. He had identified some "hot spots" in my facial area on a thermogram I had at his direction. Dr. Meyer examined me thoroughly for anything that could be causing my "hot spots." My gums were okay, he did not find cavitations (a usual culprit I am told) but he did say that I suffered from a functional mal-occlusion or bad bite.

I did not believe him at first as I have been to many dentists over the years and no one said I had anything amiss. I went away determined that it wasn't my bite. I continued to search for answers to why I didn't feel well. As last I returned to Dr. Meyer and followed his plan.

He performed some intricate biomedical tests to see how my muscles and jaw posture were functioning and out of sync with each other. He recommended and created then an oral appliance to balance my jaw. I needed to wear it all of the time. I freaked out and thought NO WAY! Well, after I got it and wore it for a few days, I realized that I no longer hurt, I was feeling better than I had felt in years. I couldn't believe it.

After some months, I began getting comments from friends that I hadn't seen for a while who commented on how much my face had changed. My face was more balanced, relaxed and actually, a nice change in my symmetry had occurred that I had contemplated having surgery to correct. It is now 3+ years since beginning treatment.

Dr. Meyer has changed my life and my appearance and I couldn't be happier. I wasn't aware of how serious my issue was, but took the chance to have the treatment undertaken. The transformation is nothing short of miraculous. I can't thank him and his staff more. I would recommend this practice to anyone searching for the best.

Conclusion

Given the nature of this book you can understand why my preferred treatments are those that are non-invasive. Always try these first, if you are deemed a good candidate. The next level up is the minimally-invasive treatments. I favor the concept of the Vampire facelift that uses your own blood derived factors that are reintroduced into your skin to give you that youthful glow. A variation of this technique that I like is the use of yet other factors from your own blood that are mixed with ozone and then reintroduced into your skin. This has the benefit of a skin filler like the pharmaceutical Restyln but is derived exclusively from you and your blood factors. The results can be phenomenal and astounding.

Use QR Code to see photo gallery of before and after:

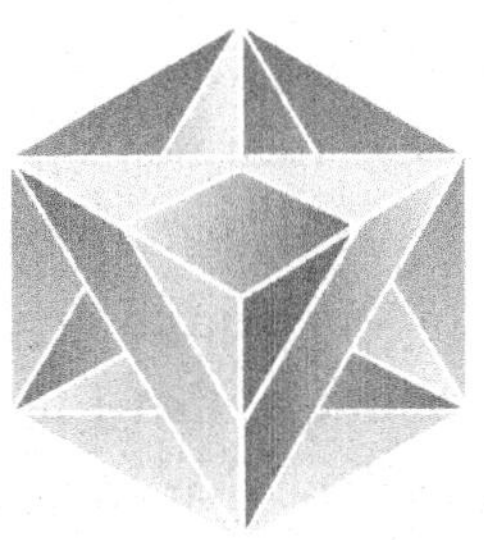

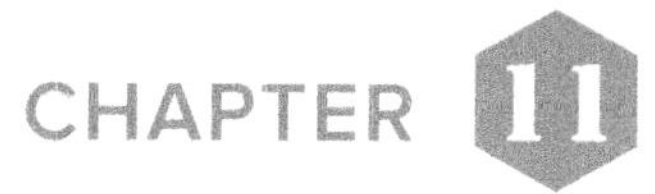

RETURN TO THE DENTAL MATRIX

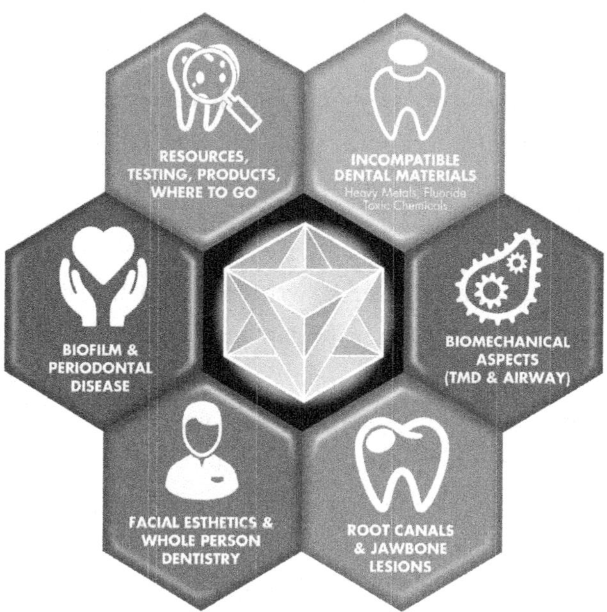

Now that you've taken a journey with me into the Holistic Dental Matrix™, hopefully you are more informed and aware of the challenges. Each of the individual chapters in this book has attempted to break down the complex nature of the Holistic Dental Matrix into manageable bite-sized pieces. This book was written for those without a deep knowledge of dentistry—or medicine. Since this is my first endeavor to share this information with a wide audience, I've used non-technical language wherever possible.

So, how do you put this all together? Well, I thought that I would illustrate the facts by giving you a few of my extended case studies. A sort of "Grand Rounds" if you will. I think it will give you some critical insight into the thought process of a holistic practitioner and help you see the wider picture.

For me, the process of understanding each piece in the puzzle starts when someone comes into my practice. In those initial minutes, I have little to go by except that the patient is usually in pain.

So first I obtain a detailed written health history from you, online via a secured service, to gather a layer of information, to increase my awareness of your particular situation. I consider this the Bronze level of information. Next we have the initial client interview which can last upwards of an hour or so. This is the Silver level where you have a pointed yet leisurely conversation with me about your situation. Often people tell me it's the longest a practitioner has ever sat and listened to them. I also read your body language, and I search your body for structural asymmetries, facial balance, tone of the speech, eye contact, etc. This is where the juice is. This is where I really start to see the picture forming of what your underlying condition or problem is. With technology as it is today, I have even performed this interview via Skype for a face-to-face virtual connection.

From here we move to an examination room for the physical examination, the Gold level. This includes: the physical counting and charting of the teeth; intra-oral photographs of the individual teeth as well as groups of teeth; an examination for gum disease with a 6 point measurement, mobility checking, recession documenting, and more; full soft tissue evaluation of the mouth tissues, throat tissues, and tissues outside of the mouth; and an orthopedic examination of the range of motion of the jaw joints as well as the neck and associated structures. Finally, I make conventional dental radiographs using high speed digital technology.

Sometimes, if your needs are limited or small in nature, you can get a plan of action right after the examination. But this occurs in only about 10 percent of the cases. Because most people have quite a complex history and physical conditions that require a bit more thought on my part, I ask you to return so we can have another conversation about the findings of the examination and discuss a course of action to treat what has been identified.

I have to tease through the multiple issues, such as those I've outlined in this book, as they intersect and come to bear on the health of each person. Behind the scenes I will usually create a spreadsheet to begin the planning process of care so that I can shift certain steps around easily as I consider each one and slot them into the treatment plan. The more disciplines that are involved, the more I need time to ponder. A discipline is an area of concern. For example, TMD, gum disease, infected teeth, cavities, missing teeth, etc.

So how do you start? Where do you go from here? How do you consider each issue? How do you come up with a plan? Those are tough questions that need good answers. I start with writing down the highlights of what you've told me and the things I've read in your health questionnaire. Then I go through a list of medical as well as dental areas that need to be checked. These are focusing tools that I use to make sure that I cover all of the bases. Fortunately I have been blessed with a curious nature that has allowed me to broaden my basic dental knowledge base.

As I go through your issues, I listen again to your story and match it against both the cases I have had in the past as well as the details of scientific papers that I have read and assembled into a library over the years. As I do that, I develop an idea of what the big picture issues are. Then I write down those next steps that can help me drill (dental humor) down into the micro details of the case.

I make every effort to gather all the diagnostic information to create or define the story in my mind. There are times, when I just have to start with something reasonable to clear away the "dust" or clutter that gets in the way that masks the situation. This is part of the process of differential diagnosis.

The following are my guiding principles when I'm interacting with a patient:

Guiding Principles in Diagnosis

1. The patient is not crazy, their malady is real.
2. Do not chase symptoms. They are guideposts to the end point, not the end point in itself.
3. Listen carefully, do not interrupt, and then ask questions for clarification to delve even deeper.
4. The emotional component of the illness must be dealt with.
5. Almost everyone has multiple layers of concerns or problems.
6. Gather enough knowledge about enough areas to "put a story together."
7. Always keep an eye out for issues involving: bad bite, gut disturbances, root canals and bio-toxins.

As I determine the issues we need to deal with, I categorize each one into Chronic, Near Term, and Acute in order to triage your care needs:

Chronic

Conditions involving toxicity, neuroadaptive behavioral mechanisms, bio-mechanical instability such as a sympathetic nervous system overload or airway collapse that leads to snoring. This also includes the downstream effects caused by your dental condition including: the trigeminal nerve complex, limbic system, reticular activating system, trigeminal nucleus, and all internal organs; acupuncture meridian energy imbalances; bio-toxin effects; and cellular/organ dysfunction.

Near Term

A combination of fewer chronic issues and some acute issues.

Acute

Conditions of recent onset including tooth pain, gum disease pain, TMD pains, etc. Also any identified conditions that will soon cause pain, bleeding or swelling.

Case Studies

The case studies I've included in this book are all true and of real people in my practice, and are used to illustrate that the elements of the Holistic Dental Matrix are real and can happen to you. These are everyday folks like you and me who have found themselves in trouble with their health and well-being because of an issue tied to their dental condition. I hope these cases do illustrate the central role that dentistry plays in your health and well-being, and that when dysfunction is missed, it can condemn the sufferer to years or even a lifetime of pain.

You can find short case studies in some of the previous chapters, but for the extended case studies below, I've supplied a narrative and a description of the treatment. Both of these stories are amazing to me because each of these individuals had suffered for years at the hands of well-meaning and well-intentioned practitioners who have had a paradigm (box) imposed on them by the traditional dental profession. Their patient's pain was within their grasp to fix, but they didn't/couldn't do anything about it.

J.

J., a 68 year old man, was desperate for relief of his prison cell of ill health. He began suffering a myriad of chronic pain symptoms after a dental procedure that was supposed to help him get better. It was a simple removal of his lower left first molar. But unbeknownst to him, this procedure led him far down the rabbit hole.

J. first contacted me on referral from a local physician in the town where he lived, after having seen at least 12 doctors in the course of about six years seeking relief. He had written out a lengthy history of both of the illnesses he had, as well as providing a plethora of medical reports from medical tests, most of which I had never heard of. We spoke on the phone through an assistant because he could not bear to have an electromagnetic signal so close to his head.

We chatted for over an hour the first time we spoke by long distance. I had him go to a local dentist to have special dental radiographs (cone beam CT scans) taken and sent to me. I reviewed the scans, but there are very few dental maladies I am aware of that can give these bizarre symptoms: body pain, cardiac arrhythmia and electromagnetic sensitivity.

Our examination checked him for a musculoskeletal condition but he was found not to have one. That left only a potential cavitation problem.

I focused on the area of my primary suspicion: the site of the removed molar. That seemed to pre-date this whole cascade of issues. When I read radiographs, I am a big proponent of looking for the symmetry of structure. Anything that is asymmetrical is worth noting. In J's case, the scan looked "funky" to me, as if there was some deformation in his lower jaw.

It appeared to me that a Neuralgia Inducing Cavitational Osteonecrosis (NICO) was located in the site where J.'s lower left first molar had been removed. To test out my theory, I injected into the site a small volume (.5cc) of non-vasoactive anesthetic that has no epinephrine. A small hole is made into the side wall of the jaw and I insert a fine needle into the hole to slowly express some fluid.

We all waited expectantly, and soon we had our answer. J. reported his pain was subsiding, and within 10 minutes, there was a complete stoppage of pain. We were all smiles. We had proof that it worked, and J. agreed the next step would be another visit to have a surgical debridement of the inside of his lower jaw.

I got a call the next day after our mini miracle and got even better news. The long-standing cardiac arrhythmia had normalized. The next call was to let me know that there was almost a full 24 hour cessation of the pain and heart arrhythmia.

That is a great result for a half cc of well-placed local anesthetic. So my next question was: When can we schedule the surgery?

Fast forward a couple of weeks. J. had the surgery without complication. I included in the surgery process the use of homeopathic remedies pre-operatively and during the procedure by injection; low level laser therapy (LLLT); saline infused with ozone for irrigation; and direct infusion of ozone gas into the sutured surgical site. His heart normalized once again and the pain was completely 100 percent gone.

I write this now after several months of continued and sustained success. It is such a joy to watch the recovery of this vibrant man. J. comes in now with the biggest smile on his face.

C.S.

C.S. is a 58 year old woman who is also from out of state. Her complaint was that she was always overwhelmingly fatigued. She had a great presence and appeared to be well-nourished and had good self-care, but fatigue was sapping her life away.

My examination process revealed that she had a small mouth, missing teeth and a root canal present on the upper right segment of her mouth in the back (a molar). I arranged to have a scan made. The physical exam revealed an absence of overt TMD issues and the X-ray was negative for an airway problem. This pretty much left the cavitation card on the table. I looked critically at the pattern (the trabecula) which is the internal architecture of the bone.

I suspected the molar with a root canal had the cavitation. Root canals can be toxic in themselves, but the resulting cavitation is much worse. The toxins are poisonous to the ability of mitochondria to create the cellular energy through the Krebs (Citric acid) cycle.

I had to go to an office in her state to perform the surgery under a complete general anesthetic. The tooth was removed along with the diseased bone. The surgery process also included the use of homeopathic remedies pre-operatively and during the procedure by injection; low level laser therapy (LLLT); saline infused with ozone for irrigation; and direct infusion of ozone gas into the sutured surgical site.

When the source of the toxin in C.S.'s body was removed, the chemical machinery of her cells could come back online and give her all of the energy that she needed. Her healing was uneventful, and she returned to the office a couple of days later and felt wonderful. She felt as if she had gotten her life back.

Empower Yourself to Wellness

Holistic dentistry can help beyond what is available in traditional dentistry because it offers "out of the box" thinking. By building on what all dentists learn in school, the holistic dentist uses a larger variety of disciplines within their practice. These disciplines cross the boundaries of Eastern philosophies and Western philosophies. We are more curious and exploratory and are less afraid to embrace concepts and technologies that make sense and work. And most importantly, we step back and look at the whole of you and consider more deeply that what we do to and for you matters on levels that go beyond just the immediate concern.

The following are testimonials from some of my patients who have realized it is up to them to empower themselves to wellness. With my help, we've been able to transform their lives.

You can hear it in their own words in these testimonials.

E.M. Testimonial

About 25 years ago I had full mouth reconstruction, state of the art for its time, to correct a lifetime of troubles with my teeth. The procedures involved lots of root canals, nickel crowns and bridges and an old style "blade" implant.

No one suspected that by the year 2014, infection slowly growing in my upper and lower jaws would weaken my immune system so much that I would develop severe eczema on my hands and arms and other skin rashes, acute irritable bowel syndrome, fatigue, fevers, Atrial fibrillation and cancer.

This was a big shock for a person who was very health oriented, active and hardly ever sick.

In March of 2014, a cancerous tumor was found in a saliva gland directly below the blade implant that held two fabricated molars in my lower right jaw. It was successfully removed and required no chemo or radiation.

I was the only one curious about why I got the cancer in my neck and so I went on a journey to discover the answer. A homeopathic M.D. in Phoenix found lots of inflamed areas in both jaws with a thermogram that suggested serious infection. He urged me to see a holistic dentist as soon as possible because such infections can lead to health issues such as cancer and heart ailments. I already had experienced the cancer.

I went to Dr. Meyer who confirmed the infections and in examining my mouth also found lots of electrical activity emanating from all the carcinogenic metal. He educated me about what the ideal treatment would be so that I could be healthy again. He skillfully and with minimal pain and recovery time, extracted all the infected root canal teeth, the blade implant, plus replaced all the nickel in my mouth with new crowns and bridges.

Six months later I can tell you that I have no more fatigue or fevers, my digestive system is greatly improved, the eczema on my hands and arms plus the strange rashes are completely gone. I am in the care of a holistic cardiologist for the Atrial fibrillation.

The cancer has not returned. Dr. Meyer has saved my life.

The problems caused by root canals and carcinogenic metals used in conventional dentistry need to be taken seriously by the medical community in order to stop the unnecessary damage to people's health.

F.R. Testimonial

I've had several tries at various anti-snore dental sleep appliances over the years with little success. However, in all the cases, I had to revert to the CPAP machine for my mild sleep apnea condition.

Quite by accident, I discovered Dr. Meyer, as my wife needed a specialist for amalgam removal. He told me things and had a higher degree of expertise that I had never heard before. I was somewhat concerned that his appliance and the cost of it might not cure my problem. I went ahead as I wanted to stop using the CPAP permanently.

The fitting, the molds taken and time spent on this were all worth it. I no longer need my CPAP machine; so I advise those affected to definitely try Dr. Meyer's solution.

K.W. Testimonial

I was referred to Dr. Meyer by my homeopathic physician. He had identified some "hot spots" in my facial area on a thermogram I had at his direction. Dr. Meyer examined me thoroughly for anything that could be causing my "hot spots." My gums were ok, he did not find cavitations (a usual culprit I am told) but he did say that I suffered from a functional mal-occlusion or bad bite.

I did not believe him at first as I have been to many dentists over the years and no one said I had anything amiss. I went away determined that it wasn't my bite. I continued to search for answers to why I didn't feel well. As last I returned to Dr. Meyer and followed his plan.

He performed some intricate biomedical tests to see how my muscles and jaw posture were functioning and out of sync with each other. He recommended and then created an oral appliance to balance my jaw. I needed to wear it all of the time. I freaked out and thought NO WAY! Well, after I got it and wore it for a few days, I realized that I no longer hurt. I was feeling better than I had felt in years. I couldn't believe it.

After some months, I began getting comments from friends that I hadn't seen for a while who commented on how much my face had changed. My face was more balanced, relaxed and actually, a nice change in my symmetry had occurred that I had contemplated having surgery to correct. It is now 3+ years since beginning treatment.

Dr. Meyer has changed my life and my appearance and I couldn't be happier. I wasn't aware of how serious my issue was, but took the chance to have the treatment undertaken. The transformation is nothing short of miraculous. I can't thank him and his staff more. I would recommend this practice to anyone searching for the best.

A.K. Testimonial

After having a root canal procedure performed, I felt there was something "off" with the tooth. I had constant pain/pressure on that side of my mouth that would radiate to my neck. I had the tooth re-examined and was told that everything was fine. Still not satisfied, I went to see a former dentist who said they could re-treat it.

Not wanting to put more burdens on my health, I researched and found Dr. Meyer. He was compassionate to my concerns.

After reaching a decision to have the tooth removed, Dr. Meyer made the whole process very stress free and for the most part pain free. I feel so blessed to have found such a kind, caring and well-informed dentist. I highly recommend Dr. Meyer and plan to continue seeing him for all of my dental needs.

My energy level is back up and I feel 100 percent better and am so amazed with the healing process that has occurred. Thank you so very much.

J.S. Testimonial

I'm writing to express my gratitude for nothing short of a miracle.

The previous state of my smile had put a damper not only on my health but on my spirit. Due to the poor choices in my early to mid-teens surrounding multiple eating disorders, a succession of teeth deterioration had occurred. And although I have fully recovered from these eating disorders and have done a complete turnaround, making health a top priority as well as counseling others in their desire to do the same; my past had resulted in the loss of three teeth and many, many cavities. Most of these cavities were at stage 4 meaning that if they were not mended then I would either be losing more teeth or undergoing root canals.

Walking into Dr. Meyer's office that day has led to one of the greatest gifts I have ever received; the gift of improved health and renewed confidence. I was previously unaware that cavities are indeed an infection in our mouths. If you look at the tooth/body correspondence chart (the Dental Health Matrix), you will see that these mouth infections (cavities) affect multiple body systems which compromise our health and balance. Left alone, ultimately cavities can lead to disease. For someone who is so attentive to health and balance, this was rather unsettling. Also, I had two previous amalgam (mercury) fillings. I was aware of the detriment these cause to our bodies but had not found a qualified person I was comfortable with to take these out. Dr. Meyer's removal process was foolproof and now I am proud to say that my mouth is mercury-free.

The care that I received in Dr. Meyer's office was that of family; from the receptionist to the hygienist to the doctor himself. I felt very safe and comfortable. I was thoroughly listened to and understood, allowing me to overcome my fear of dentistry knowing I was in capable caring hands. The previous state of my mouth was obviously horrific, however I had feared the overwhelming procedures, costs and inadequate or detrimental care I may receive going into just any dental office. What drew me to Dr. Meyer was that he is a holistic dentist, meaning that he takes the entire body into consideration when working on the mouth and teeth. And after meeting him in the initial consultation, I finally felt comfortable committing to healing my mouth.

That commitment led to an incredible, life-changing experience and a miraculous gift. When I came back for the results of my exam, I was informed that I had been chosen for a scholarship to fix my teeth! I am still in shock and awe. In just two days I went from being infected with cavities, unable to confidently smile and laugh… to a flawless grin. I now can smile and laugh without worrying about revealing unsightly teeth. What was once a dream is now reality thanks to Dr. Meyer. I highly recommend him and am forever grateful.

H.T. Testimonial

My first visit at Millennium Dental was to visit Dr. Meyer regarding mild sleep apnea. He had suggested a custom fit mouthpiece and it worked beautifully. No more problems regarding that situation.

I remarked to him how self-conscious I was about my smile and I had teeth that were misaligned. I confided in him how upsetting it was but I did not want to wear braces.

Dr. Meyer changed my life. He redesigned my smile and bite with veneers and they look so beautiful. People tell me every day what a perfect smile I have. I never wanted to smile before. My appreciation is beyond words and he has restored my mouth and I will be forever grateful to him and his expert knowledge of dentistry.

K.S. Testimonial

I sincerely thank you for your excellent help. Since the oral surgery, my health is dramatically improved! I'm so happy to tell you that I haven't felt this well in years. I'm deeply grateful to you for all you've done for me.

A.C. Testimonial

I am very happy with the bite correction work I had done by Dr. Meyer. He helped me to better understand how my dysfunctional bite was affecting the rest of my body. I had been so accustomed to moving my jaw forward, backward, left, right in order to bite, chew, etc., that I did not notice how overworked my neck muscles were and how this made it difficult to relax my neck to fall asleep.

I had had braces three times and was aware I had overbite and overjet issues and had been told the only way to truly correct my bite was to have jaw surgery to extend my jaw forward, yet I had not taken that drastic step. I was pleased to learn from Dr. Meyer that he could achieve better function for me non-surgically and that the process would include removing my amalgam fillings. I have a degree in biomechanics and could both understand and experience for myself the biomechanical validity of Dr. Meyer's diagnostic steps and corrective procedure, so I decided to let him work his magic. My whole body has always been hyper-mobile, and as I age, my focus in exercise has become stability, to better control my mobility. Having a jaw that could not find a stable home was likely not helping the stability of my pelvis.

I am quite pleased with my outcome and appreciate the efficiency of my chewing. I no longer have to have a tug of war to take a bite from a stick of celery or remove a bite of fibrous food from my mouth because I can't chew it sufficiently. When I lie down to try to sleep, my neck muscles can relax because my teeth engage in such a way that my jaw naturally stays in place, instead of floating or having to "land" in a non-central location. I am also pleased with the aesthetic outcome, as my jaw sits a bit further forward than it used to, and now my teeth have veneers (to achieve a color match for the material added to bite surfaces to improve my bite). Throughout the several month process, Dr. Meyer explained each step, and he and his staff were very pleasant to work with. Thank you, Dr. Meyer!

Below for a video testimonial of a very complex medical-dental condition:

Conclusion

After reading these case studies, I hope it is very evident that there is a significant emotional component to the Holistic Dental Matrix. You see, dental problems transcend the domains of the physical, emotional, mental, spiritual and etheric. This interwoven fabric known as a "human" has these very real domain issues touching all areas of their lives and being. I am humbled to know that I touch some of the most intimate aspects of one's being in the work I do. When I began my journey in dentistry a bit over 40 years ago, I had absolutely no idea this is what God had in store for me.

I hope this book has given some hope to those who are searching for answers to their woes. Sometimes the path becomes obvious and direct while at other times it is winding and circuitous. If you have hung in with me through the end of this book my guess is that you have one of the more circuitous journeys to navigate. I honor your journey, however far and however long it may be.

NAMASTE

CHAPTER 12

HOW DO I GET HELP?

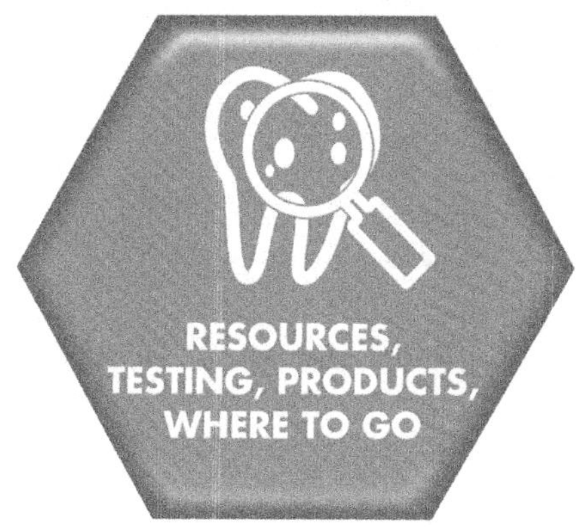

Here, in this final section, I'd like to give you some of the organizations that exist in the U.S. that can help you with various elements of the Holistic Dental Matrix. If you have been with me from the beginning, congratulations! You will be well rewarded for your efforts in having better health and well-being for either yourself or a loved one.

Not all of the listed organizations encompass all of the topics presented within this book. Not all of the organizations' members have the same or even equivalent qualifications. As there is no specialty for this area of special interest, there is no uniformity of training nor credentialing.

This is where you'll need to do additional homework. Some of the organizations are somewhat single-discipline focused. That is, they have a focus on only one aspect of the Matrix. The first three listed, in my opinion, can offer you the closest to a one stop practitioner. However, you must satisfy yourself that the doctor is going to be the right one for you and verify that their qualifications match as close as possible to the needs you have.

Organizations

Helpful Dental Organizations

International Academy of Biological Dentistry & Medicine - IABDM.org

International Academy of Oral Medicine and Toxicology - IAOMT.org

Holistic Dental Association - HolisticDental.com

Academy of Biomimetic Dentistry - AcademyofBiomimeticDent.org

American Academy of Physiological Medicine & Dentistry - AAPMD.org

American Academy of Craniofacial Pain - AACP.org

International Academy of Physiologic Aesthetics - TheIAPA.com

American Academy Clinical Sleep Disorders Disciplines - AACSDD.org

American Academy of Oral Systemic Health - AAOSH.org

American Sleep and Breathing Academy Dental Division - ASBAdental.com

Mercury Safe Dentists: www.mercurysafedentists.com

Helpful Medical Organizations

Arizona Homeopathic & Integrative Medical Association - Arizona Homeopath.org

Sacred Medical Order of the Church of Hope - SMOCH.org

American College for Advancement in Medicine - ACAM.org

Academy of Integrative Health & Medicine - AIHM.org

American Association of Naturopathic Physicians - Naturopathic.org

Pastoral Medical Association - PMAI.org

Veterinary Organizations

American Holistic Veterinary Medical Association - AHVMA.org

Support Materials

Blood Serum Compatibility Test Kit – Bio Comp Laboratory: www.biocomplaboratories.com. There is a fee to have the blood drawn as well as for the test.

Definition of Terms

The following pieces of equipment and terms have been used within this book. They are presented here again for a more complete and thorough definition, as used within these pages. I do not believe that you will find them at odds with any other use.

Diagnostic Devices

Bio Impedance Analysis (BIA)

This technique is made possible by several different device manufacturers. The device measures a variety of physiological parameters. Often you will find personal trainers using one of these devices during an initial assessment. One parameter is used for the body's ability to heal by holding an energy charge in the cell membrane. This is determined by what is known as the Phase Angle.

Cavitat®

Medical ultrasound that has been used both diagnostically and therapeutically for decades. This adaptation of the diagnostic version yields information about the health of the bone of the jaw. We are looking for areas of ischemia harbored within the jaw bone. The display is one of a three dimensional cube of bone volume. It displays almost a tooth-by-tooth look, much like a dental X-ray.

Cone Beam Computerized Tomography (CBCT)

This is a three-dimensional CT scan of the jaws and adjacent structures. Your doctor uses this to look at the relationships of the various structures to compare them. Depending on the type of unit your doctor has, there may be additional benefits of a CT scan. These include seeing the size of the airway passages and the sinuses, as well as measuring bone architecture to see if there is adequate volume of bone for dental implants (when needed). Not all dental CBCT units are created equal nor are their software interfaces readily useable from one doctor to another. It is akin to translating between Spanish, French and Latin. Similar but way different.

AMA (Acupuncture Meridian Assessment)

This is a device that assesses the flow of energy within the body as measured by points along acupuncture meridians on the hands and feet. Some devices are simple in nature and require the operator to introduce test substances into the circuit, while others are integrated with a computer and these have digital signatures of substances that can be tested for you.

K-7®

This is a suite of instruments that gives real time measurement of the movement of the jaw and the muscles through time and space. It allows us to measure postural position, muscle activity, internal jaw joint integrity and more. This is used in advanced diagnosis of TMD issues, compromised bite relationships, airway analysis, etc.

Pharyngometer®

This is a device that measures the oral/throat airway passage. This is used both diagnostically and for treatment modulation. The device emits sound waves that strike the structures in the mouth and throat and then are bounced back to a microphone in the device. The computer interprets the wave pattern and displays it as a two-dimensional representation on screen along with three-dimensional numerical values of the various sizes of certain openings.

Rhinometer®

Related to the Pharyngometer, this device works similarly but on the nasal passages. It sends sound waves through the external nostrils to the back of the throat and the bounce-back is interpreted by the computer. We are looking for blocks from the shelves inside the nose (turbinates). Often the airway problem is in the nose and not the throat (as is often assumed). This gives us the window to peer into this structure.

Treatment Devices & Procedures

Anodyne®

This is a low level laser therapy delivery device that aids in the "up regulation" of the healing process by increasing nitric oxide within the cells receiving the energy. It is applied immediately after surgery for 30 minutes. There are instances that this device will be used for a more prolonged basis such as the treatment of shingles. It carries FDA approval for the treatment of neuropathy. It is also known as Monochromatic Infrared Energy (MIRE™).

Bio-modulator®

This micro-current device is a diagnostic instrument as well as a treatment device. It is used for a plethora of conditions including bone healing, anti-inflammatory action and pain relief. Coupled with the companion bio-transducer, subtle energy can be delivered deep within the tissues where surface stimulation just cannot reach efficiently.

Extractions

All of our tooth removal procedures are deemed surgical in nature. In addition to the removal of the tooth, the periodontal ligament is removed along with any diseased tissue. Supplemental adjuncts include: lasers (LLLT & High energy), ozone, homeopathic remedies, PRP, PRF, etc.

Bone Grafting

This is a bone enhancing procedure where atrophy has already diminished the volume of the bone. The donor bone can be from one's self (autograft) or from another source (xenograft). The choice of which to use is made based on need (volume) and location.

Homeopathic Remedies

An old healing discipline with the premise: like treats like. Holistic practitioners use a variety of homeopathic remedies to support your body in detoxification and healing. A remedy is administered either via sublingual drops or injectable form.

LANAP

A patented technique that stands for Laser Assisted New Attachment Procedure that uses a specific kind of laser to remove diseased tissue, sparing the healthier tissue. Also usually involved is cleaning the roots of the teeth and then bite adjustments.

Lasers

I use two different types of lasers in the management of gum disease. They have differing wavelengths and thus a different tissue reaction. Lasers all work with light that is one color and one color alone. This is called monochromatic light and is coherent (all waves are traveling in the same direction). The light from a regular light bulb is chaotic and non-coherent.

Lateral Ridge Augmentation

This assists your body to "grow bone" on the side of a jaw that is deficient in width. Most commonly found in the lower jaw and the front part of the upper jaw.

Mill Calm

A unique blend of the following: neurotransmitters, brain synchronizing music; cranial electrical stimulation (CES) and visual field blockade. This results in a brain state that is in harmony and optimized for rapid relaxation. Used together they induce a deep alpha brainwave state within five minutes. The result is a very calm, comfortable dental visit for you.

Microbaric Ozone Insufflation Therapy

The delivery of life-giving oxygen through the use of ozone gas. Ozone is applied to the gum tissues by means of both direct injection into the tissue or through delivery by a cannula (a tiny tube) into a void or defect in the between the gum and tooth. It can also be delivered through the creation of a custom system of specially designed trays that deliver ozone gas through a closed direct pressure system to the whole arch at one time.

Ozonated Irrigation

Ozonated saline is super-charged saline that is used to irrigate or wash a site to bring energy deep within the tissues that have just had a surgery. It provides the antibacterial effects inherent with ozone.

Sinus "Lift"

This procedure thickens or enhances the bone volume between the floor of the sinus and the "ridge" to allow for the placement of a dental implant.

Socket Preservation

This treatment is done at the time of the removal of a tooth to maintain as much bone as possible in a tooth socket. Socket rebuilding is used when the tooth socket walls have been damaged and need bulk to allow for the placement of an implant.

Soft Tissue Procedures

There are a number of procedures that are used to enhance the soft tissue of your mouth. These procedures can be done strictly for cosmetic reasons or to assist in the functional needs of an area that is being contemplated for a graft. This includes free gingival, a soft tissue procedure to gain additional "attached" tissue. Also connective tissue, a soft tissue procedure to thicken or bulk up lost tissue.

EPILOGUE

It was serendipity that put me on an airplane next to Nancy Meyer, Dr. Nicholas Meyer's wife. She told me that he was writing a book on holistic dentistry and was looking for an editor. When she explained his theory that our teeth are connected to the other parts of our bodies, I understood where she was coming from. I've had successful holistic medical treatments in the past, such as acupuncture to aid in fertility, and I consult regularly with a Naturopathic Doctor who advises me on nutrition, cleansing and supplements.

With my background in publishing, I knew I could help Dr. Meyer produce his book. But in order to fully understand his Holistic Dental Matrix, I had to try it for myself. So I went in to see Dr. Meyer at Millennium Dental Associates for a consultation. From the first minute, I was really impressed with his practice and the people in his employ. From the ambiance to the care, it was a soothing, thoughtful experience.

First Dr. Meyer took a detailed written health history from me that was much more in depth than anything a dentist has ever asked for before. Then we had a consultation where we sat down at a table in his office to discuss the health issues that were bothering me. I thought it was a wonderful way to begin. It made me realize that the only time I've ever spoken to a dentist is when I'm already lying on my back in the dental chair. Dr. Meyer's consultation, on the other hand, made me feel as if time was truly being taken to learn about me and what I felt my body needs.

Then Dr. Meyer gave me a physical exam. Since X-rays of my teeth had been taken within the past two years, he was able to use those instead of subjecting me to additional radiation. But he did take intra-oral photographs of each of my teeth using a tiny camera. He was able to zoom in very close and project the image on a large screen mounted on the wall to show my teeth. I could see where the teeth with mercury fillings were cracked, while the ones without silver fillings were sound and whole.

It was eye-opening to be able to see my own teeth in such magnification. But the exam was just beginning. Dr. Meyer counted and charted my teeth; probed for gum disease; performed mobility checking; did a soft tissue evaluation of my mouth, throat and lips; and an orthopedic examination of the range of motion of my jaw joints as well as my neck.

It was the most thorough exam I'd ever had in a dental office. After it was over, I went back to sit down with Dr. Meyer face-to-face to find out the results. As I already knew, I had mercury fillings that needed to be removed before they continued to damage my teeth and my health.

He told me that the mercury fillings had caused several of my teeth to crack, in particular my back right molar in my lower jaw.

That molar had a large crack down the back side that I could see in the image. When that molar was wiggled, it moved quite a bit and was very painful. I realized that tooth had been aching for quite some time but I just accommodated by chewing on the other side of my mouth and avoiding that area.

Dr. Meyer's advice was to have that lower molar removed ASAP. Dr. Meyer gave me three different kinds of homeopathic medicine to assist in healing from surgery: one which helped my body's natural cleansing process of lymphatic drainage; another which is used to aid in recovery from surgery; and lastly, one which is a drainage remedy for relief of general congestion to flush the toxins from my system.

Dr. Meyer also told me that my bite was misaligned. He asked me if any dentist had told me that I have an overbite. I said no. But when I looked at my teeth, I could see that my front teeth completely overlapped my bottom teeth. It felt as if my teeth came together and meshed well that way.

But Dr. Meyer said it was a problem. My tongue was pressed very hard up against my front teeth. It was crammed into my mouth which made it hard to breathe with my mouth closed. It was also deforming the bones of my jaw. I had developed a ridge above my right upper mandible because my upper teeth had been forced upward due to the pressure from my lower molars.

Dr. Meyer asked me to say the word, "Yes" with a sibilant hiss. He told me that was the "neutral position" for my jaw. In the neutral position, my lower jaw moved forward so my teeth met end-to-end. That left a gap between my back teeth. I felt my jaw relax and move forward, but it also made my cracked molar throb in pain even though there was nothing touching it.

Putting my jaw into that position was so difficult that it felt wrong, but at the same time, it felt very right. I tried to hold that position for as long as I could, and it felt as if the muscles in my face were relaxing in my cheeks and around my eyes and between my brows on my forehead. I've always had a deep "11" between my brows, and I could feel the tension there easing and my eyes opening up. I realized the amount of tension I had been holding in my jaw was incredible. I almost couldn't force myself to relax, and the pain from my molar was so bad that it keep me awake all night.

The main reason I persisted in saying "Yes" to put my jaw into the neutral position was because I could finally breathe that way. The back of my throat opened up when my lower jaw moved forward. I suddenly had a rich flow of air, and I felt almost euphoric in spite of the pain.

That morning before I went to see Dr. Meyer to get my back molar pulled, I looked at myself in the mirror. I could only move my jaw forward somewhat because of the pain, so my teeth weren't meeting end to end. They were still overlapping despite my best efforts because of that right rear molar.

I went in for surgery and the molar was in such bad shape that it came out with hardly any effort by Dr. Meyer. It was apparently the lynchpin of my mouth because with that molar gone, it felt like my jaw could finally relax and move forward where it belonged. My teeth now meet end-to-end. In spite of the surgery, my face felt better. My tongue was able to lie flat in the crescent of my mouth.

There was very little pain from the hole where my molar was extracted—*unless* my jaw clenched back into an overbite. When I deliberately tried to overlap my front teeth to make my old bite, I couldn't because the pain where the molar used to be was too extreme and I was afraid of ripping the stitch out.

By the second day after surgery, I could already see a difference in my face. It looked longer and my eyes were more opened up. My mouth saw the biggest change as my bottom lip looks fuller and new dimples formed at the corners of my mouth. I realized all of my features looked kind of squished before, and now they've eased.

On the third day, I felt an intense ache on the upper right side of my jaw where my teeth were no longer clenched together. It was like the nerves were relieved of the constant pressure yet couldn't stop firing in phantom pain. The boney shelf above those upper back teeth throbbed. I wondered if that shelf will slowly collapse now that it's not being shoved up into my cheek by my bottom molars.

By the fourth day after surgery, there was pain radiating all the way up to my ear from the release of pressure on the right side of my jaw. I could also feel my Eustachian tube open up on that side, and when I breathed, I felt air passing through. The pressure in my ear kept breaking as well. It felt much looser in my jaw under my right ear compared to the left side.

The phantom pain eventually went away. Now when I do deliberately try to clench my teeth in an overbite, I can feel where my teeth ground against each other for years because they're more sensitive there. On the other hand, my front teeth had to get used to tapping together because that's never happened to them before.

I also had to get used to the different way my tongue feels. It now rubs against my teeth on the back along my molars instead of along the front. The serrations on the front of my tongue, where my teeth used to leave little indents, have faded away.

Now my jaw feels much looser and has a larger range of motion. I try not to chew the way I used to, but as it turns out, I used to chew very far forward because there was no room to chew in the back. Now I can chew further back because my teeth don't meet anymore. I didn't realize you could chew between teeth that don't grind together, but it works well for me now. But at first, I felt a bit like a two year old learning how to chew again, and I had to think of every bite.

It would have been harder to maintain this new jaw position but for two things. First, breathing is wonderful and I can now get nice, full breaths with my mouth closed. Second, in the beginning whenever my jaw pulled back by habit, the pain from where my rear molar was extracted alerted me that I was grinding my teeth and over-biting again. I was able to consciously form the new habit of holding my jaw in the neutral position by relaxing the muscles in my face.

I feel very fortunate that I met Dr. Meyer. He's the dentist who has explained my overbite. With the removal of that rear molar, I was in the perfect position to take advantage of his knowledge and help heal damage that has gone on for decades. It's shocking that my previous dentists never told me that I had an overbite that should be corrected. And it's amazing that pulling a tooth could help shift my jaw forward so dramatically. No wonder that molar cracked—my body wanted that tooth out!

Now it's very natural for my jaw to rest in the neutral position. Even when I wake up, it's that way. My eyes have opened up bigger. Not only can I feel it, but I can see an edge of white under my pupils which I never saw before. And my chin is more pronounced.

The day after Dr. Meyer removed that molar, in spite of the surgery, I felt such a pervasive feeling of well-being that I was astonished. In fact, the glands under my armpits had been swollen and sore off and on for many months, yet my doctors couldn't find any reason for this reaction. After the molar was removed, the random swelling in my glands stopped completely.

I had spent the year before the molar was removed spontaneously questioning myself as I was falling asleep at night, wondering "Am I okay?" But I'm no longer doing that. I think the slowly growing pain from my molar was alerting me subconsciously that something was terribly wrong.

I had told Dr. Meyer in our initial consultation about that bad feeling I kept having as I was falling asleep at night. That's not something I would ever tell a dentist as he was leaning over me ready to look into my mouth. But Dr. Meyer's focus on the entire person, a holistic way of treating your health, created the space for me to share what was really happening with me. He listened and understood. That opened the path for me to reach true healing through his treatment.

Today, I'm looking forward to getting the rest of my mercury fillings removed properly by Dr. Meyer, and having a more beneficial treatment for my dental issues in his hands. I hope that you get as much from this book as I got in helping Dr. Meyer publish it.

INDEX

Symptoms, Chapter

Made in the USA
Coppell, TX
18 January 2021

48366181R00164